Arthritis—
Stop Suffering, Start Moving

ARTHRITIS— STOP SUFFERING, START MOVING

DARLENE COHEN

Illustrations by Susan Aldridge

Walker and Company
New York

First published in the United States of America in 1995 by Walker
Publishing Company, Inc.
Published simultaneously in Canada by Thomas Allen & Son Canada,
Limited, Markham, Ontario

Library of Congress Cataloging-in-Publication Data
Cohen, Darlene.
    Arthritis—stop suffering, start moving / Darlene Cohen.
        p.   cm.
    Includes bibliographical references and index.
    ISBN 0-8027-1308-4.—ISBN 0-8027-7466-0 (pbk.)
    1. Arthritis—Exercise therapy.   I. Title.
RC933.C63   1995
616.7′2206—dc20
                                              94-45682
                                                CIP

Book design by Susan Hood

Printed in the United States of America

10   9   8   7   6   5   4   3   2   1

Contents

Acknowledgments

I will always be grateful to my teacher, Meir Schneider, not only for encouraging me as a student, but for transforming my life.

For their support, care, wisdom, friendship, and example, I wish to thank David Chadwick, Carol Harris, Beth Bebout, Daya Goldschlag, Elizabeth Sawyer, Linda Ruth Cutts, Peter van der Sterre, Blanche and Lou Hartman, Michael Wenger, Iva Jones, and the Bodhisattvas at the San Francisco Zen Center who got me through the worst of it.

I rarely get a chance to heap public praise upon my husband, so I would like to take this opportunity to bring attention to his many excellent qualities, notably his wit and humor, his generous and unstinting support, and his determination to make love to me under adverse circumstances. For this and much more, I thank you, Tony Patchell.

Ethan, thank you for your patience.

D.C.
San Francisco
January 16, 1995

Preface

One of the most fundamental observations I have made as a movement teacher for people with arthritis and spine problems is that when movement hurts people, they usually stop moving. This of course creates a degenerative situation—strength and mobility are lost over time. When we have difficulty moving, we need to learn how to use movement itself to decrease rather than increase the pain by substituting healing movement for motions that cause strain and stress. This book will teach you healing movement, thereby helping you regain lost mobility. Believe it or not, you also will learn to take pleasure in movement.

When I developed rheumatoid arthritis, I was a relatively young woman living on a somewhat isolated farm in Marin County. I had never had any contact with anyone suffering a debilitating physical injury or dis-

ease. I knew only strong, young, healthy people. As I became increasingly helpless and crippled, I was devastated emotionally as well as physically.

Conventional avenues of remedy did not help me. The options I was given for relief (an array of drugs ranging from somewhat toxic to very toxic, to be taken the rest of my life) added to my sense of hopelessness. I called the Arthritis Foundation for advice, hoping the staff could suggest alternative treatments or inform me of some innovative research programs. They said to follow my doctor's orders, that there was nothing beyond what he had told me. They were very concerned that I not become the victim of any of the multitude of quacks out there looking for desperate people like me to prey upon. They kindly sent me a catalog of prosthetic devices that would enable me to put on clothes and reach things without moving very much. Of course, everyone meant to be helpful, but I found this passive, function-without-movement approach very discouraging. *I wanted to move again.* I wanted to find a way to reconstruct a real life for myself out of the hobbled remnants of the old one.

Eighteen years later the choices I made then have been vindicated by research showing that exercise is of primary importance to arthritis sufferers, that the drugs used to treat arthritis symptoms (cortisone derivatives and nonsteroidal anti-inflammatory drugs) weaken bone tissue and increase the incidence of ulcers. The Arthritis Foundation now offers its own exercise program in warm pools all over the United States. Yet with some notable exceptions (Dr. Dean Edell and various self-care magazines edited by physicians), people are still encouraged to take a passive role with regard to their own well-being and health. For the most part, we are not made aware of the tremendous healing resource we have in our own bodies, in our own conscious awareness of our activity. For whatever reason, we still tend to rely primarily on external remedies for pain and restricted movement instead of exploiting our own enormous potential for expanding our wisdom and cultivating good health.

I wrote this book to tell you there is a lot you can do for yourself that you may not learn in the institutions of conventional medicine. And you don't have to take my word for it either! You can get the necessary information from your own body. Once you learn to trust the feedback you get from your body, you won't be confused over questions about diet, exercise, pain relief, and activity level, nor will you have to worry that someone else has given you the wrong advice. The healing powers of your own body provide the ultimate in safe and natural therapy for arthritis.

The best news is that your daily life itself can be the key to your healing if you live it in a manner that incorporates the information that your body is always giving you. The way you get out of bed, the way you walk, the way you work and enjoy yourself—all these motions and activities can make you stronger and more whole. This book is intended as an instruction manual for converting your daily life into an effective twenty-four-hour-a-day treatment plan for your disease. By incorporating your whole being and everyday activities into this plan, you can transform your life to an extent you might not have thought possible.

Part I

OUTSMARTING ARTHRITIS

Chapter 1

The Self-Healing of Arthritis: My Own Story

I first began to suffer the symptoms of arthritis in 1977, when I was thirty-five years old. Until then I was a very active and energetic person, enjoying hiking over the coastal headlands and walking on the beach near my home in northern California. I also studied Japanese tea ceremony, which is an ancient, highly ritualized, and very subtle celebration of time, space, and social graciousness. It involves sitting still upon the knees for about three hours at a time. This position is painful after a while, but as soon as one stands up, the pain disappears. My first arthritis symptom presented itself after a long session of kneeling; I stood up, and the pain remained. I could hardly leave the room. It took more than two hours for my legs to stop hurting and return to normal.

A few days later, upon getting back from my weekly hike, my knees and ankles were so swollen and painful that I had to lie down for several hours before resuming normal movement. Stairs became increasingly difficult even if I hadn't hiked recently. My hands started aching, and they weakened to the point where I couldn't manipulate scissors or a can opener. I woke up in the night with pains in my neck and hips. I lost my appetite and began to lose a lot of weight. Finally, as the pain and then the fear increased, I went to a physician and was diagnosed as having rheumatoid arthritis.

The visit to the physician that day was the beginning of the worst period of my life. He told me I could start taking anti-inflammatory drugs to alleviate pain and swelling. I would start with the least toxic drug, and if that did not work, I would try increasingly more toxic drugs, which he would monitor closely. Every patient was different, he said, and there was no telling which drugs would work or what side effects would occur until we tried them. The physician assured me that I had a number of options, including surgery for the joints that had already been damaged. He emphasized that there was no cure.

I went home from this meeting extremely depressed. I was trapped in my body. I lay on my bed and alternately wished for a miraculous intervention or the simple relief of unconsciousness. I just could not accept this condition. I had been a vital, unusually energetic woman. I had a two-year-old son and a demanding job that I loved. I liked challenges; I liked finding creative solutions to difficult problems. Now everything was swept away. I couldn't work; I couldn't play; I couldn't even hug my son without feeling pain wherever his body pressed against mine. I lay in bed and watched the sun set from my bedroom window.

I thought a lot about what the doctor had said about taking anti-inflammatory drugs. What it boiled down to was that relief was a possibility, but toxicity was a certainty. Maybe my symptoms would be alleviated and maybe not. In either case, the drugs would not cure me. The warriors of my immune system would still continue to attack healthy cells, believing for some unknown reason that the synovial fluid around my joints harbored an enemy. There was appar-ently no way to derail the arthritic process at the source by correcting this inappropriate immunological response.

I decided I was too young to begin relying on a lifelong drug therapy to treat my arthritis. In subsequent years I would make that same decision again and again.

There was also some part of me, defeated though I was, that wanted to stay in touch with and learn to control what was happening to me. Outwardly, I had become extremely passive because of the pain that accompanied every movement. Inside myself, I had the idea, rough and as yet unformed, that I would have to find my own way through this. Someone else, somewhere, must have gone through this, and I could, too. I needed a clue, a starting point.

In dealing with this catastrophe, I was fortunate in a number of ways. For one, I lived in a community of people who shared a common purpose, the study of zen meditation. I had friends who took care of me and my son, and so I never had to go to a hospital. People dressed me, cooked for me, cleaned the two small rooms of the little house my son and I shared, and did our laundry. I was oblivious then, preoccupied with my pain, but now I realize how lucky I was that people were willing to care for me and that they did so in such kind and affectionate ways. Friends and acquaintances came to me with all sorts of remedies. Some would bake wheat-free bread for me. Others brought me herbs and wrapped me in comfrey-soaked sheets. Still others took me to acupuncture treatments. Friends gave me wonderful massages, poured me tea, and took my son for days and weeks at a time. But despite all this care, I continued to deteriorate.

Now all my joints had become affected: my feet, ankles, wrists, and fingers. My spine began to curve at the neck so that I stood stooped over as if I had spent my life working in rice paddies. The pain was unceasing and overwhelming. It hurt too much to prepare food and eat; I had gradually lost thirty pounds. I finally became so weak I couldn't tolerate having people around me at all. My memories of that time are of lying in bed and studying the patterns of the sheets and blankets. Restlessness merely drew my eye to the paint chipped around the windowsill. This was stimulation enough, because I had no energy at all. Four long months had passed. I was in a vegetative state, and my miraculous intervention was long overdue.

At about this time a well-meaning friend came by with a catalog of prosthetic devices, clever little aids one could purchase to help everyday functioning. There were devices for pulling on socks, buttoning blouses, and clothing with Velcro enclosures that eliminated the button/zipper problem altogether. This catalog forced me to face, finally and undeniably, that my illness was not going to go away by itself. Here was proof on page after page that there were many people in the world who would never again pull on their socks or button their blouses unaided. After my friend left, all the dormant feelings of rage and bitterness rose up through my despair to protest. I could not, would not, live like this!

All along, friends had been telling me about Meir Schneider, an intense young man from Israel who worked with desperate cases such as mine in a converted storefront on Taraval Street in San Francisco. He had been born legally blind—barely able to distinguish light from dark—and had brought himself into the sighted world by developing what little vision he had. Ignoring the professionals who had told him he would never see, he began to do eye exercises in his teens. He went on to develop his vision to the point where he could read, and recently he had even earned a California's driver's license. Friends of mine had gone to see him: one with a bad back, another with a pinched nerve, and a third with multiple sclerosis. He began working with all disorders in the same general way: by relaxing his clients and then guiding them to sense in their bodies the same minute discriminations that he had found pivotal in developing his vision. Through the process of sensing and moving, they were able to discover and develop their bodies' own healing potential. That appealed to me. I called Meir and made an appointment to see him.

At first my pain proved a great barrier to

treatment. I was sullen and passive. I couldn't stand to be touched, and I shrank from Meir's fingers. Because I also couldn't bear to move, I refused to do the prescribed exercises. My body felt like a closed, dense, heavy cage. I felt restriction in my chest every time I breathed. I was surprised when Meir encouraged me to feel my restrictions, rather than deny them. He told me I had to start by actively immersing myself in my current suffering instead of holding it from me with painkillers and fantasies of waking up the next morning miraculously well. He told me to give my physical pain my full attention by locating it in specific parts of my body; to admit the extent of my immobility and the motions I could no longer do; and finally, to accept the feelings of anguish that accompanied this frank acknowledgment of my loss. Only by starting with this much awareness could I get access to the information that would alter my suffering.

I also was fortunate that I had been studying zen for a number years, and I understood exactly what Meir was advising me to do. The practice of zen meditation is to observe one's own bodily sensations, thoughts and perceptions, and emotional feelings as they occur. When you meditate on these events, you aren't trying to change them. You simply recognize that you are standing or sitting; you are intensely aware that you are thinking about what you will be doing later in the day; or that you are hearing cars passing outside

or feeling a little anxious, and so on. You notice your internal and external environment. There is no goal involved.

The practice of self-healing, on the other hand, is to make these same observations and then to manipulate the sensations, thoughts, perceptions, and feelings that you are able to observe in order to improve your health. Since I had a background in zen, it was not difficult for me to continue to make these observations in the service of my healing.

It was true; by focusing on my actual bodily sensations, I began to find the smallest movements here and there, places in my body that were neither paralyzed nor painful. I discovered a tiny movement in my chest that I could make without pain, so for the first time in many months I could enjoy breathing. That place was such a refuge, such a joy, I returned to it again and again, like a cat lying in a favorite spot in the sun. I found that I could move my thighs together and apart when I lay on my back. I delighted in feeling these small and precious spaces in my fossilized body and then enlarging them, spreading them into other restricted areas of my body. It was a powerful experience for me.

Meir Schneider taught me many small movements. I do not mean "exercises" such as those we tend to think of when we think of exercises: "twenty to the left, twenty to the right." They were more like meditations on movement, movements that develop body awareness. If you pay attention to *how* it feels to move a certain way, you begin to sense your body's yearning for motion. It will tell you quite specifically what it wishes you to do, and your movement begins to be determined by your body itself. Start with any motion—small, slow ones are best—and simply *feel* your body doing each tiny part of the motion. You begin to learn what your body needs and what it wants to do next. By following my body in this way, I began to open paralyzed places. I found that if I could make the motion small enough, there was no paralysis in my body. Those parts of me that were impervious to feeling or movement from the inside became, eventually, wonderfully responsive to the touch of my own hand.

The exercises I did were very gentle: hip rotations, ankle rotations, finger, wrist, and neck rotations, some back bending, and lots of rubbing of my fingers and knees. I followed the line of pain to its source. During my daily exercise sessions I concentrated on each part of my body for a short time; then I did overall stretching and bending. First, I massaged an area to bring in blood and cell nourishment. I moved the joint gently, then vigorously, and I synchronized these movements with my breathing in and out. For those times when I was just too tired to move, I lay on my bed and imagined my body expanding as I breathed in and contracting as I breathed out.

And so I began to recover. A year later I could once again cut with scissors and lift pans off the stove. I resumed working full-time, and I gained back the weight I had lost. Vitality flowed back into my body. My son could hug me once again without my shrinking from his embrace. I was walking with a noticeable limp but without pain. Someone gave my son a small toy robot. He wound it up and put it on the floor. "Look!" he cried, delighted. "It walks just like you, Mom!"

I was impatient to be totally normal again. The progress I made was accompanied by tremendous frustration. I would work for weeks on a particular area of my body without any improvement at all, and suddenly that part would break free and I would be encouraged to continue once more. Then there would be no progress for weeks. Many times I thought I was being foolish for not just taking arthritis drugs; it would require so little effort compared to what I was doing. At that time I didn't know other people with arthritis, and I assumed the drugs would be at least as effective as my exercises.

One particular day I had just finished doing my exercises, the usual series I had been doing for some time to try to reduce my limp: hip rotations, swinging my legs back and forth, stretching each leg out behind me, touching my toes while my leg was outstretched on the table. After I finished, I left my house to meet a friend. It was a sunny day, and the air was crisp. As I walked I got looser and looser, and when I saw my friend in the distance, I suddenly felt the urge to run. I began running toward him, laughing and crying; such a thing had been unthinkable for two years! Similar experiences periodically affirmed my path for me.

As part of my exercise program, I began going every morning to the heated pool at the San Francisco Recreation Center for the Handicapped. There I did more complicated large muscle movements to strengthen my body, movements that would have hurt me on land. I met many people with arthritis at the pool, and I discovered that I was the only one who didn't take some sort of drug for pain or inflammation. Astonishingly, though, I realized I had originally been in worse shape than all but one of my fellow swimmers, yet I was now the most mobile of anyone there! I became very impressed with my good fortune and stopped doubting my path. Within a short time I was asked to teach my exercises to others in a weekly class at the recreation center.

I had learned a great deal about pain and movement over the course of my recovery. Recognizing this, Meir Schneider asked me repeatedly to join him in his work with chronically ill people. He understood before I did what a storehouse of information about arthritis my body had become and how useful it might be to others. At first I resisted, perhaps because the memory of my suffering was still too close and I wanted it all far behind me. But as my appreciation of my body's healing powers grew, as my energy and joy increased, and especially as my friends and then their friends came to me with their own difficulties, I found myself drawn to teaching what I had discovered. I became fascinated with the individual differences between people and the individual means by which healing powers are created and evoked.

In 1980, three years after I was first stricken with rheumatoid arthritis, I began training and apprenticing with Meir Schneider. I worked with him on a variety of degenerative conditions and came to know people who faced what I had faced. These were people who could reach beyond their despair to help themselves by drawing on their own inner resources.

I have been working with such people for fifteen years now. I teach classes in movement and give lectures on self-healing. I hold arthritis workshops in which we do the movements that are basic to daily activities: dressing and grooming, cooking and housework, walking and going up and down stairs, getting up from a chair, and driving a car. I recently completed a fifty-five-minute video on which four of my clients and I demonstrate the gentle movements that have helped to ease painful symptoms and restore function to our arthritic joints.

I participated in a bike marathon last year

and regularly go whitewater rafting in northern California and Colorado. My life, which fifteen years ago seemed to be over, is now full and rich. I strongly encourage other people who feel overwhelmed by their pain and restriction to seek healing within their own bodies. This can be done. I am just one among many individuals who can testify to the innate resiliency and creativity that is part of the human body. We need only dare to look for that space, regardless of how small, where movement resides and recovery begins.

Chapter 2

Challenge and Release: The Paradigm for Healing Arthritis

To start healing your arthritis, you must understand and apply the principle of challenge/release, whereby the nervous system, muscles, or joints are challenged—that is, activated by a demand—and then released. A good example is a step. When you step down on your foot, you are challenging your toe, ankle, knee, and hip joints, as well as all the muscles and nerves that attach to them. When you pick up that foot again, all the joints, muscles, and nerves that were stressed are now relieved. When you put that foot down again, you can feel the pressure, the stress, the activation of your entire lower body. When you pick your foot up again, your lower body is released, and so forth, over and over again. Thus, walking is a good illustration of the challenge/release paradigm

and an ideal exercise for people who are able to walk without pain.

Exercises that incorporate this principle are excellent for arthritis because they challenge the joint just enough to keep it strong and functional, and then release the joint in time to prevent injury or pain. Rapid alternation of challenge/release is also very effective in reducing the chronic swelling of arthritis. For example, here is a good exercise for joints that are swollen but not very painful: Get on your hands and knees, which immediately puts pressure on the swollen area of your knees. When you move your torso forward toward your hands and backward toward your heels, the pressure on your knees is alternately increased, then decreased.

If joints are very painful, the pressure

should be applied briefly and lightly. Instead of getting on your hands and knees, you might lie on your stomach and rotate your calves and feet around your knees with your feet in the air. Another example of brief, light pressure is that of lightly and briskly stamping painful feet on a bed or carpeted floor. This rapid alternation of pressure and release reduces swelling and prepares sore feet for the body's weight.

The challenge/release paradigm is applicable on many levels: to stimulate individual body parts, to reduce swelling, and to gauge rest periods. People with arthritis know that the best way to plan their days and weeks is to follow challenging tasks with periods of rest. It is counterproductive to attempt to spend most waking hours completing difficult chores. You get sore, exhausted, and discouraged. Nor does it feel good to lie around most of the time, to do only simple tasks, and to leave most work to other people. Your joints and muscles deteriorate, and you lose your energy, not to mention your will to live.

It is important to find a balance between challenge and release that is best for you at different times, that takes into account that you feel energetic sometimes, lethargic at other times.

It is hard to learn to pace yourself. When you feel good, it seems natural to want to push, to get those things done that you've let slide during less comfortable times, and it's easy to end up doing too much. However, once you have become familiar with your own basic energy patterns (daily peaks and valleys); once you know from doing the exercises in this book which parts of your body are likely to tire first and become dependent on which other parts; once you have tuned in to the subtle cues by which your own body indicates whether what you are doing right now is increasing or depleting your energy— then you have begun to participate in the wisdom that your body has to offer you, to receive information from it about what is helping it or hurting it at all times.

You can learn to trust your body's mes-

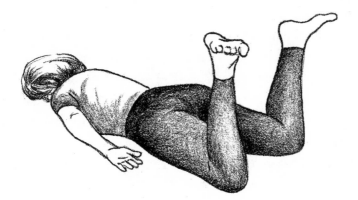

sages. You will come to know what is completely comfortable and what is questionable. You will see that some activities leave you quite tired but refreshed the next day. You will learn which activities cost too much— afterward you will feel terrible for at least a day. This is an extremely useful ability to develop: a totally reliable internal mechanism you can count on for the information you need in order to plan your activities. It is difficult to overcome your desire to get things done according to an abstract (non-body-oriented) schedule, but you must put aside this desire in order to be able to receive your body's messages.

The importance of body wisdom and its superiority to abstract thought for healing was brought home to me early in my struggle with arthritis. My therapist had given me a series of water exercises to loosen my contracted body and to give me a light feeling I couldn't experience on land. I faithfully went to the warm pool and did what he told me: I spent an hour raising and lowering my legs in the water, spreading my arms out away from my chest, rotating my ankles, and gently turning my body from side to side in the water. These were extremely effective movements; I always got out of the pool feeling loose, light, and pain-free. But every day while doing my gentle exercises, I watched people who could swim back and forth doing laps. After some weeks I began to resent my

"sissy" exercises and envied the swimmers their grace and strength.

Finally my envy accumulated to the point where one day I abandoned my exercises and attempted to swim like the others. But my weak, tight body refused to make the motions necessary to pull myself along smoothly in the water. Instead of feeling refreshed and loose when I got out of the pool, I felt sore and exhausted. I tried this several more days before feeling so terrible that I gave up and sadly resigned myself to my gentle little movements.

After three more months of doing my exercises faithfully, I began to feel energy rise within me and to feel discernibly stronger whenever I came out of the water. Gradually I began to notice that my exercises made me a little restless. It became clear to me that my body wanted a greater challenge. One day I felt compelled to jump off the floor of the pool and glide through the water. I swam from one end of the pool to the other and back again. I was thrilled; my body felt to me like a single, agile unit firmly moving me through the resistance of the water. I swam lap after lap until I felt tired. When I got out of the pool, my heart was beating, my muscles were throbbing, and my spirits were high. My body itself had yearned to swim. The yearning had not been an impulse arising from denial and envy; the desire to move came from my viscera, from my muscles themselves. That experience at the pool taught me resoundingly that my own body is the irrefutable judge of which challenges I may take on, not imitating other people or making intellectual decisions.

Accepting a challenge that you *can* meet does several things for you, physically and psychologically. It makes you stronger in the sense that you have expanded your behavioral repertoire. Your mind's idea of yourself is wider and not only includes the specific behavior you just exhibited but is now more open in general to the possibility that you will successfully meet another challenge. This is how your mind and body expand infinitely. Your brain learns that there is some boundless aspect to you, some heretofore undiscovered and unimagined facet of your abilities. The preconceived restrictions begin to fade. I believe this kind of triumph has a biochemical concomitant in the brain that influences the release of hormones and neuropeptides that strengthen the immune system and reduce pain.

The importance I place on including challenging activity in a life dedicated to healing comes from my own experiences of somehow transcending my arthritis when I am moved beyond my usual boundaries by some enrapturing physical adventure. Let me elaborate on what I mean by this. Normally, day to day, I live *with* my arthritis. We share the same body. I'm aware of stiffness, some hesi-

tation in my joints, whenever I change my position from sitting to standing or quicken my pace to catch a bus or dance several dances and then sit down. Because of that awareness, I'm always slightly stretching with each movement. It's second nature to move so that I create a subtle stretch in various joints, which gives me the gratifying feeling that I have plenty of space in which to move my body. This is how I live with arthritis. It is a very good adjustment to a degenerative disease. However, when I've accepted a certain kind of challenge, one that exhilarates me, that tests not only my bones and muscles but my ideas of what I as an arthritic person can do, I feel some kind of "systemic override." I don't know whether what I feel is based in physiology, but I do feel as if some other healthier, unfettered aspect of my body has been released and has overcome the arthritis. I'm no longer an arthritic, cleverly maneuvering around my stiffness; I feel actually free: No motion I do will call up the hesitation, the shadow of constraint that routinely accompanies my change of posture. I feel as if I no longer have arthritis!

For instance, I felt this way the first time I went whitewater rafting. I had wanted to go on a rafting trip for some time but was afraid I was too weak, that I would get hurt or might hold up the group, or that something else unforeseen but embarrassing would occur. Finally, after thinking about this activity again and again, I found myself calling up and making reservations. I asked a friend with arthritis to go with me so we would have each other. She canceled the day before, but I was too excited to turn back. Full of doubts and fears, I sucked in my breath and drove alone to the river. It was a very hot day. I looked at the cool, gently rolling river with its little whitecaps. I said hi to the other people. I got in the raft.

I was happy as we glided downstream, my lifejacket snug against me, the river gorges jutting up into the sky around me, the water playing with the one foot I had thrown over the side of the raft. Then the guide announced our first rapid coming up. I pulled my foot in and readied my paddle. The waves grabbed our raft and tossed it among the rocks. While I screamed, my muscles applied themselves to the paddle; my back and legs rode the current as if it were a horse. Safe again in the gentle current, I laughed and laughed. Five hours later, back on the beach, I was drenched, sun-tanned, filthy, and ready to sleep. I was also deliriously happy, even ecstatic. I knew my body well; I could feel its deep strength and pleasure-induced sense of well-being. Impulsively I signed up for another trip the next day and found a motel for the night. After a shower, I fell asleep immediately, a smile on my face.

The next morning I had the feeling that arthritis had left my body. I met my group and took another ride down that exhilarating river. Driving home tired and happy that night, I encountered a sudden thunderstorm, which lasted about ten minutes. I opened all the car windows and felt the fresh cold water on my muddy, sweaty skin. For nearly a month after that trip, I felt no arthritis. It gradually came back as my normal life continued. But I had made an important observation: I realized for the first time the great significance of pleasure/ecstasy in healing.

Another time I decided to sign up for a thirty-mile bicycle marathon. I had been feeling good for some months, and my usual fifteen- to twenty-mile rides no longer satisfied my physical yearning to ride until I was very tired. The route of the marathon went through some of the most beautiful parks and gardens south of San Francisco, and raised money for arthritis research, so I signed up. I was rather nervous, both about the distance and about needing to commit myself ahead of time, but I figured I could just leave the event whenever I got too tired. Thirty miles of splendid scenery later, I was still going strong. I was tired, but feeling exhilarated from my accomplishment. I had enjoyed the route so much, with its profusion of flowers and spectacular views, and I had been able to feel my chest, shoulders, hips, and legs loosen as I rode. When I got off my bike at the end of the race, I tested my joints for soreness by moving them in subtle ways the biking did not include. Despite my demanding day on the bike, they felt great.

Again, I emphasize that these were challenges that arose from my body itself. They were born of a restlessness and yearning to move that I could feel. They did not originate in my head, with my envy of others' abilities or with some abstract wish to prove what I could do to deny my disease. *When the desire to meet a challenge arises from your body, the very activity that would ordinarily tax you and make you weaker makes you stronger.*

A client told me the following case in point: She was home alone on a Saturday morning, planning to go out later to do some shopping. She had promised herself, however, that she would do a few gentle exercises for a while before going out, in accordance with her instructions from me. The problem was that she didn't feel like doing any exercises. She felt restless, agitated, not at all in the state of mind conducive to lying down on the floor and doing meditative movements. As a matter of fact, she felt rebellious about the whole thing. She looked at her piano and thought about how she had wanted to move that piano into another room for a long time but had never done it because she knew such a strenuous task would further injure her already strained back.

She thought about moving the piano now, in the way I had instructed her to move generally: using her arms and legs to make any exertion, bringing her back into play only after her arms and legs were fully engaged and active. She went over to the piano and

began to move it. It took her nearly an hour, but she moved that piano into the other room, little by little, carefully checking that her arms and legs were fully engaged at all times. Not only did she not injure her back, but she felt exhilarated and much stronger and looser after moving the piano than before. It was her body's restlessness—its yearning—that she had heeded.

In taking on challenges meant to raise my capacity, I have made mistakes. Once I signed up for a ten-day dance workshop that promised individual pacing. I felt that my body yearned to experience this rhythmic movement requiring strength in the same way I had yearned to glide through the water. I had been doing my own small movements alone for some time, and I needed some greater challenges. Once at the workshop, however, I strived to keep up with the younger, more energetic women who not only danced all day but partied into the night. I felt like going to bed after dinner, but I ignored my bodily sensations in order to satisfy another need, that of being included in the social life of the participants. By the end of the workshop, the arthritic feelings that had been overriden at the beginning had returned in full force. I was exhausted. I stayed in bed the morning of the last day, sore and miserable. After I got back home, I was barely functional for a couple of days. Experiences like this have taught me to give the deep feelings from my body the greatest attention and to meet whatever other needs I may have with whatever is left over. I have learned that *no* needs get met unless I feel physically energetic and pain-free.

Challenging Your Body When You Feel Very Low

As you sit at the window in a painful body, you look out and watch others walk, run, play, or show evidence of their vitality. You know it is emotionally devastating to compare yourself to others. You must return your mind to this moment, your own body, your own present level of movement, and make your thoughts and sensations your whole world right now. Rest assured that however little movement you are capable of now, you *can* increase it a little and feel you are making progress. If your whole body aches, do something that brings some ease and energy to it. Breathe slowly and deeply into your diaphragm, and bring the breath up into your chest so that there is some movement in your upper body. As you sit, lift first one foot, then the other, a few inches off the floor so that your lower body and feet feel a little more active. Do the movement in a slow, rhythmic way that is comforting and enjoyable. Let the sensations arising from your body's movement fill your consciousness. *At times like these, your own world must be compelling enough to sustain you through your envy of others' abilities.* The more physical satisfaction

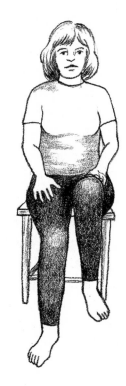

you can evoke from your body at this time, in your own way, with your own accomplishments (getting dinner, going to the bathroom, being self-sufficient), the easier it will be for you to avoid the pitfalls of comparing yourself to others. You can push aside your envy and depression and feel a resurgence of your own energy.

Techniques to Challenge Your Body at the Most Restricted Level

Whenever you reside in a painful, barely functional body, first assess what your body *can* do. What are your restrictions? Where is your pain worst? Gently and patiently, begin to soften the edges of your restrictions by slowly easing into them with small movements that reduce your pain. Here are a few techniques to get you started.

Your Fingers

If you can barely move, merely lie down, or sit down, and quietly feel the breath going in and out of your body. Open and close your hands so slowly, with such awareness, that you can feel the heat of your fingers as they approach your palm and feel the coolness of the air as your fingers leave your palm. If this movement is painful for your fingers, bend and extend one finger at a time, so slowly and so precisely that it doesn't hurt. Follow the rhythm of your breathing, inhaling as you flex each finger and exhaling when you release.

Your Shoulders and Neck

While you're lying down or sitting in a chair, raise and lower each shoulder, one at a time, in the same rhythm as your breathing. After you have been moving your shoulders long enough for them to feel easier to move, stop moving your shoulders and slowly begin to move your head from side to side. Move your head very gently so that it moves freely with no effort on top of your neck. Feel as if someone has your chin in his hands and is gently moving your head from side to side very slowly. Alternate this movement with your shoulder movements. Open and close your

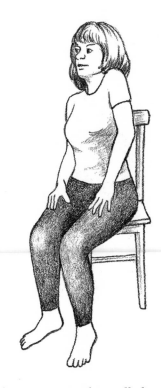

hands. If you can, combine all these movements. Doing all these movements at once will make you feel looser, more flexible, more capable of movement. If you stay well within your range of motion, not straining to your limits, your brain will register that you are moving without restriction, and you will feel free.

Your Lower Body

Sit with legs comfortably apart. Keeping your feet where they are on the floor, gently move your knees toward each other, then back. The rhythm of this movement should imitate that of your breathing.

If you are lying in bed, bend your knees

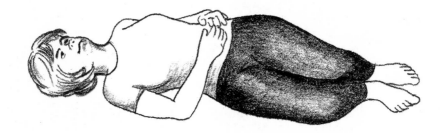

with your legs and feet together. Relax your hips and belly, and slowly move your knees from side to side. Keep the knee movement gentle enough so that you have no pain. Your knees are touching each other, your feet are close together, and your knees move gently across the midline of your body, first to the left and then to the right. Whenever you exhale begin to move your knees to the other side of your body.

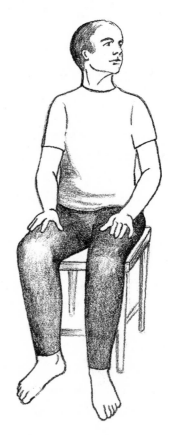

Benefits for Your Body

Whether sitting or lying, moving parts of your body slowly, gently, and without pain lets you feel the mobility of your body; you begin to appreciate your body's capacity, as it is in this moment. Your body is your whole world at this moment. Within that world of sensation and movement, you can improve. You can enjoy movement. You can accomplish something.

At the end of a movement session, it is possible for you to get up feeling as refreshed and accomplished as someone who runs a marathon race. It is not easy to run a race; but it is also not simple to open up a painful, limited body. Both endeavors are accomplishments to be proud of.

Applying Challenge and Release to Your Work

As we have seen, being heedful of the challenge/release paradigm means alternating vigorous activity with periods of rest, or no effort. This principle can be applied as well to two different activities; you can alternate an activity requiring one kind of effort with one requiring another kind of effort. For instance, walk for a while, then sit on a bench and stretch your upper body over your lower body before getting up and continuing the walk. Swim vigorously with the body pushing through the water, then float idly, letting the water move your body. Pedal your bike up a rise, then pedal backward as you coast down the other side.

You can divide any task into periods of effort and relief. By doing so, you are able to vary the stimulation you receive and stay at the task longer because you are getting rest periods while doing the task itself. You can push the vacuum cleaner across the carpet, then relax your muscles as it cleans in one spot, then push it again. You can push your shopping cart down the aisle, then pull it backward to retrieve a particular item. While gardening, you can work on your knees, then work from a seated position. When you brush your hair, you can lower your arm at the end of a stroke, then raise it again. When you put dishes away in the cupboard, the effort is raising your arms to the shelves; the release is letting your arms fall to your sides before picking up some more dishes.

A carpenter came to me as a client because her back hurt constantly during her work. She recovered partially on days off and completely during extended vacations, but as soon as she returned to work, her back would start to hurt again. I suggested that she become very conscious of the specific demands her work made on her body. She was to notice which work tasks required her whole body to make an effort (e.g., when she carried heavy tools or lumber from one place to another) and which tasks required only certain parts of her body to become actively engaged (e.g., when she fitted two joints together or hammered nails). Once she had this new awareness, she was to relax the parts of her body that were not directly needed for a given task. After following this advice for a few weeks, she found her back problems had almost completely disappeared, and she had much more stamina. She had learned when to make an effort and when to release her body, instead of tensing her whole body all the time. The constant, unrelenting application of the muscles to a task with no interval of relief is what tires you and makes your work period unsatisfying.

Alternating Challenge and Release in the Same Movement

The principle of challenge/release, or effort/relief, can also be applied to a single movement. In the simple motion of rotating your straight arm around your shoulder, for example, there is a point of maximum effort, minimum effort, and relief from effort. When you begin to lift your arm, to pull it away from gravity, you need to make a great deal of effort. At the top of the rotation, when your arm is straight up from your body and your hand is pointing toward the sky, effort is still required, although less is needed than for the initial motion. When you begin to let your arm fall, the more synchronized with gravity your arm's angle becomes, the less effort is required to move it. So you experience some relief, until you lift your arm against gravity again. Similarly, when you lie on your back and move your knees from side to side with your feet close together, you will notice that you must make an effort to begin to move your knees from one side to the other. But when your knees are in motion and falling to the other side, you feel relief, not effort. Inhaling usually requires more effort than exhaling. To maximize your vigor, make a conscious and deliberate distinction between effort and relief as you perform your daily activities.

Chapter 3

Arthritis and the Whole Person: Body and Mind

People usually think of arthritis treatment as targeting only the joint that aches. But the healing of arthritis also requires that a person take steps to support the functioning of the various systems of the body. Care has to be taken to raise the level of general health. The relative emphasis given to systemic health and joint repair depends on the type of arthritis and the damage already sustained by the joints. All forms of arthritis are systemic to the extent that tissue health and pain level are affected by circulation, inflammation, and the amount of oxygen in the blood, but some forms, such as rheumatoid arthritis, gout, and lupus, are the direct result of immune system dysfunction and are therefore very much affected by changes in overall health. In general, however, this chapter will be useful for all arthritis sufferers. Guidelines for working on joints are provided in chapter 4.

Some key factors that aid systemic function include emotional influences: attitudes and emotional states, a feeling of control, the pursuit of pleasure, nurturing relationships—as well as proper diet, movement, and breathing techniques. Let's examine each of these in turn.

Emotional Influences

Emotional States Influence the Immune Response

The immune system is currently the most heavily researched area in medicine, in large part because of the AIDS crisis. It is now believed that the course of many diseases may be dramatically affected by the so-called mind-body interactions, with their biochemical basis in the immune system. A new medical discipline called psychoneuroimmunology has sprung up to study the mind-body connection. For years, health professionals have observed that patients with a "positive" attitude seem to recover more easily from serious illness. We've all heard of someone whose disease went into remission after the person got involved in a new romantic relationship, took up meditation, went on an extended vacation, or whatever. Now medical research is turning up scientific evidence demonstrating how the release of hormones and endorphins, the brain's natural opiates, affects the functioning of the immune system.

Dr. Candace Pert, a visiting professor at the Center for Molecular and Behavioral Neuroscience at Rutgers University, calls it an "astounding revelation" that "these endorphins and other chemicals like them are found not just in the brain, but in the immune system, the endocrine system, and throughout the body. These molecules are involved in a psychosomatic communication network. . . . Everything in your body is being run by these messenger molecules, many of which are peptides. . . . We've actually found the material manifestation of emotions in these peptides and their receptors. These receptors floating around on the surface of the cells put out their little antennae and re-

ceive what's coming in . . . viruses use these same receptors to enter into a cell, and depending on how much of the . . . natural peptide for that receptor is around, the virus will have an easier or a harder time getting into the cell. So our emotional state will affect whether we'll get sick from the same loading dose of a virus. . . . Emotional fluctuations and emotional status directly influence the probability that the organism will get sick or be well."[1]

Dr. Margaret Kemeny, a medical psychologist at the University of California in Los Angeles, studied patients with genital herpes with regard to their stressful life experiences and took blood samples from them every month for six months. She found that those who were depressed suffered significantly more recurrences of their herpes lesions than the others in the study, and their blood tests also showed a significant decrease in the number of T cells, a type of white blood cell that attacks foreign invaders and thereby helps provide immunity.[2] Discussing her research on the relationship between emotions and the immune system, she told Bill Moyers during their interview for his *Healing and the Mind* series: "There may also be some adaptive physiological consequences to experi-

[1]Candace Pert, "The Chemical Communicators," (interview) Bill Moyers, *Healing and the Mind* (New York: Doubleday, 1993), pp. 178–79, 190.
[2]Margaret Kemeny, as reported in *Medical Self-Care*, January/February 1989, p. 31.

encing emotions. States like depression, which don't allow us to experience our emotions fully in response to the environment, may have a different impact. When we're depressed, we often are less responsive to the environment emotionally. There's certainly accumulating data now that chronic depression has negative biological consequences as well as psychological ones."[3]

Kathleen Dillon demonstrated a link between positive emotional states and enhanced immune function. Students who viewed a humorous videotape had significantly higher levels of salivary immunoglobulin A—a type of antibody that appears to defend against viral infections of the upper respiratory tract—than controls who watched a didactic tape.[4]

In a study led by J. Stephen Heisel of Charles River Hospital in Wellesley, Massachusetts, it was noted that the "healthier" a research subject's personality, as measured by the Minnesota Multiphasic Personality Inventory (MMPI), the more laboratory cancer cells were killed by the subject's white blood cells.[5] On the MMPI, a healthy personality combines tolerance, confidence, and self-esteem. A high depression score, on the other hand, indicates a person inclined to withdrawal, guilt, low self-esteem, and fatigue. Those who ranked high on the depression scale had less active killer cells. Other researchers at the University of Michigan found that volunteer work dramatically increased life expectancy in men. In trying to explain such results, stress researchers hypothesized that the feelings of warmth and well-being from doing good were the factor responsible for prolonging life. Endorphin production apparently contributes to feelings of well-being.[6]

Because of the startling (to the medical world) findings of much of this research, indicating the importance of attitude and emotion to health, it is important to consider this aspect of our healing when we must live with a degenerative disease.

A Feeling of Control

The extent to which an individual can exercise control over his or her life has a profound effect on physical as well as mental health. This effect has been seen in the laboratory during a study of rats who had electric shocks applied to their tails. Those rats who were unable to end the shocks not only exhibited many signs of depression, such as poor eating and no interest in sex, but also showed major changes in

[3]Margaret Kemeny, "Emotions and the Immune System," (interview) Bill Moyers, *Healing and the Mind* (New York: Doubleday, 1993), pp. 202–3.

[4]K. M. Dillon, B. Minchoff, and K. H. Baker, "Positive Emotional States and Enhancement of the Immune System," *International Journal of Psychiatry in Medicine,* vol. 15 (1985–86), pp. 13–17.

[5]J. Stephen Heisel, as reported in *Hippocrates,* July/ August 1987, p. 88.

[6]James House, as reported in *American Health Magazine.*

their immune systems, such as a dramatic drop in the number of their white blood cells. Another group of rats, who could end the shocks by turning a wheel in their cages, showed no such signs of depression or drop in white blood cells. The psychologists performing this study called the depressed rats' condition "learned helplessness."[7]

Many epidemiologists believe that the same thing happens to human workers when they must perform jobs that have negative stress built into them. Scientists believe the factor responsible for the built-in stress in such jobs is a feeling of loss of control. Workers are given wide responsibilities combined with a lack of personal control over how work is done. When the relationship between this kind of job stress and serious health problems like hypertension and heart attacks was explored at Cornell University Medical Center, researchers found that these workers were at least four times more likely to have hypertension than those with all other types of jobs.

People who develop a degenerative disease also experience "loss of control" with reference to their health and the functioning of their bodies. Their first realization is that they can no longer order their bodies around as they once were able to. In the arthritis

workshops I have held, people talk most about their loss of control, the betrayal of their bodies. This seems to be a major issue for people with serious illness. Since the research cited above suggests that patients' feelings about being in or out of control are a *health* issue as well as a psychological one, it is important that a sense of control be restored as soon as possible.

Deciding to take responsibility for one's own health, rather than passively handing it over to a health-care practitioner, has been linked with a lessening of symptoms. In a series of experiments conducted at the Stanford Arthritis Center, an arthritis self-management course was designed to help patients with arthritis cope better by teaching them exercises and self-care. Compared with a control group, the participants exhibited significantly less pain. However, surprisingly, the people who improved were not necessarily the ones who demonstrated that they had learned the most or most often engaged in the therapeutic exercise. The key difference between those who improved and those who did not appeared to be the person's perception of his or her own ability to control or change the arthritis symptoms. This quality the researchers termed "self-efficacy." When the self-management classes were reorganized to maximize this sense of self-efficacy (by modeling successful coping behavior and providing specific skills), there was a significant correlation

[7]Steven F. Maier and M. Laudenslager, "Stress and Health: Exploring the Links," *Psychology Today*, August 1985, pp. 44–49.

between improvements in symptoms and perceived self-efficacy.[8]

It would appear that making the decision to heal one's self is crucial for anyone with a systemic illness. From my experience with my own body and from observation of people I teach, I have come to believe that there does seem to be some biochemical concomitant of active, conscious, deliberate attempts to heal one's self. Practicing relaxation techniques seems very important, perhaps because they enable the individual to pick up on the body's signals through the garble of goal-oriented thoughts, panic over one's condition, and pragmatic advice from others. This is not to say that I am against consultation and treatment from physicians. I just think it is not conducive to one's health to become passively dependent on *anyone*.

Cortisone injections, exercise classes, or massage take place a few hours a week and have an immediate physical effect lasting probably a few hours to a few days. If your therapy accounts for only a few hours out of a possible 168 hours a week, that leaves well over 100 hours when you aren't doing much for yourself. (And even if a person had the resources to afford to have several hours of therapy a day, the regimen would not evoke the critical biochemical response if he or she passively accepted therapy.)

When you feel in control of your physical mobility and your pain level, even a flare-up of your disease will have less impact on you than on someone who is dependent on "fate" or another person for his or her ease. You know that you can work through any setback or recover any temporarily lost function. A person in a victim stance, by contrast, will be overwhelmed by fear and panic, further aggravating an already toxic system. According to a study published in 1983 by Marvin Zuckerman of the University of Delaware, some of the rewards for accepting a physical challenge are feelings of mastery, competence, confidence, strength, endurance, knowledge, self-control, and the empowering feeling of overcoming fear. As Dr. Zuckerman concluded, "Our biochemicals may influence what we feel like doing, but what we do also influences our biochemicals."[9]

The Relentless Pursuit of Pleasure

When people ask me for some instruction on how to manage their pain, I answer very emphatically that they must begin immediately to commit themselves to the relentless pursuit of pleasure. Usually people are surprised

[8]K. Lorig, J. Laurin, and H. Holman, "Arthritis Self-management: A Study of the Effectiveness of a Patient Education for the Elderly," as reported in *The Healing Brain,* by R. Ornstein and D. Sobel (New York: Simon and Schuster, 1987), pp. 247–48.

[9]M. Zuckerman, as reported in *Vogue,* September 1988, p. 520.

to hear this advice. But I really do mean the *relentless* pursuit of pleasure. A wishy-washy pursuit of pleasure does no good because it implies you are willing to experience pleasure only if it wanders by after other more important things are out of the way. Don't let yourself get bogged down by chores and obligations. They must be secondary to the most important thing: your enjoyment of life. Pleasure and laughter and a sense of life being worthwhile have biochemical implications for your healing that must be given primary importance if you are serious about healing yourself. For many people, giving pleasure this kind of priority is not easy since most of us have been brought up to consider other people first and to perform our perfunctory duties before seeking pleasure. Sometimes, however, for the sake of your health, you have to break your old habits—especially if those habits have compromised your health in the first place.

The first time I ever noticed this pleasure-healing connection, I was sick with active rheumatoid arthritis, and I was very sensitive to different kinds of food. Wine and sweets seemed to attack me with particular ferocity. An hour or so after drinking wine with dinner or eating some favorite sweet, I would be in agony, my joints screaming with sharp pain and my whole body aching as if my blood itself had needles in it. So of course I almost never indulged in these former treats.

One spectacularly beautiful day some friends took me with them to the Point Reyes Seashore to have a picnic. It was very kind of them to include me since it was not easy for them to transport me and all of our food and equipment to the beach. But it was one of those golden days when everything works out. They placed me on a blanket by the shimmering ocean, and I breathed the sea air and felt the warm sun on my skin with great pleasure. I watched the waves as they crashed onto the beach and the kids and dogs playing on the shore. I felt relaxed and happy. When the food, including cookies and pie, was spread on a blanket and left out for the group to nibble on all afternoon, I partook freely of the bounty. When the wine was passed around, I drank some, feeling expansive and unwilling to deny myself any pleasure.

Later, after we had gathered our things and driven back to San Francisco at twilight, I suddenly realized I hadn't felt the pain usually associated with drinking alcohol and eating sweets. In fact, I actually felt better than I usually did at the end of a normal day of dragging my reluctant body around to perform its necessary functions. I fell asleep immediately after getting home. When I woke up the next morning, I felt better than I had in months.

This experience made a deep impression on me. I thought a lot about it. I had taken into my body a great deal of what my body treated as poison. But in this instance it either hadn't recognized the food and wine as poison in the first place or had disposed of it efficiently. Why? I might have been so relaxed that perhaps my hormones, enzymes, and digestive juices were secreted in the proper proportions by glands that were not compressed and inhibited by pain and contraction. Maybe my body had just undergone normal digestion for a change. Or possibly my bodily processes were positively influenced by endorphin production. Under conditions of deep relaxation and pleasure, the nervous system secretes neuropeptides, which influence the functioning of the endocrine and immune systems. Perhaps pleasure activates these systems to function more efficiently. Perhaps it merely inhibits the production of "stress hormones" or produces a decreased responsiveness to major stress hormones that may inhibit digestion. However it works, pleasure puts my arthritis into remission, sometimes for only a day, other times for months on end.

Physicians may dismiss this phenomenon as another instance of the placebo effect (improvement in one's condition because one believes one is recovering), but I believe that the so-called placebo effect may be a major aspect of healing in *all* situations and that without it, very little healing of any consequence takes place. I think that patients actually allow their doctors and therapists to heal them in accordance with their expectations and belief systems. They go into the

therapy situation expecting healing and ultimately *permitting* healing. Perhaps the mechanism behind the placebo effect is the mind-body interaction, discussed earlier in this chapter. As Dr. Herbert Benson, director of the Division of Behavioral Medicine at New England Deaconess Hospital, concludes in his book on the relaxation response, "The power of the mind over the body may . . . encompass many medical problems that we have tried to treat only through physical means or perhaps have regarded as medically untreatable."[10]

A feeling of well-being is the most important consideration in this book, besides movement. If you ignore everything else I recommend or describe, you can probably make considerable gains on your illness by seriously pursuing pleasure and gently moving your body.

Nurturing Relationships

WITH THE BODY AND INNER SELF.   Most of us, normal and active since childhood, are unprepared emotionally to face the loss of mobility. Especially in this culture, where our bodies are the slaves of our mind-constructs, we pay little heed to the needs of our bodies in most circumstances. We are almost always involved in carrying out some mental plan we have devised. Thus the refusal of my

[10]Herbert Benson, *The Relaxation Response* (New York: William Morrow, 1975).

body to carry out these plans was a great shock to me—a mighty betrayal by a servant who, without provocation, had deserted me and would not be moved by the urgency of my pursuits and demands.

People who have experienced this betrayal must acknowledge the strong feelings of despair and bereavement that surround it. Because we tend to view these feelings as not "rational," in the sense that it is not particularly helpful at such a difficult time to blame our body itself for our misery, some people suppress these feelings or fail to acknowledge them fully. But it is to our great benefit to deal with them directly, to process them in some way that clears our body of these hard feelings.

Without this acknowledgment, we may harbor unhealthy anger, conscious or unconscious. Sometimes people even hit themselves or slap the areas of their bodies that refuse to work properly, as if the offending parts were acting out of some perverse, spiteful obstinacy.

It is important to accept these difficult feelings as part of the process of getting well. For me, it helped to think of my body as a neglected child who could not go on any longer without love and attention. This image came to me when I was first ill, spending most of my time lying in bed, alternately sleeping and lying awake. Sometimes it seemed to me that some internal little girl

was speaking to me, begging me for attention. She was thin, obviously neglected, and in a desperate emotional state. She begged me to take care of her, to nurture and love her. Today in psychological circles much is made of the child in us, the one who is left to starve while the adult "planner" monopolizes the organism. For me, acknowledging the anguish and repairing the emotional damage that this forgotten child was experiencing became an important aspect of my healing.

Even if no "inner child" beseeches you, it still may be a good idea for you to assume that there is some part of you that would benefit from your kind attention, some part of you that you've been neglecting in your goal-oriented world. Perhaps you have resolved to hold to a lifestyle that demands the capitulation of your body; you're continuing to subject your body to a set of rigorous demands. Maybe you have imposed a healing program on your body with the same ruthless fanaticism with which you forced yourself through your daily schedule before you became ill. Such actions may seem justifiable in terms of the hostility you feel toward a body that has let you down. It is useful to explore these complex feelings with a support group or a private therapist when you are ready to focus your attention on your healing.

Perhaps the most important aspect of your

relationship with your inner self is learning to nurture yourself. This means learning to appreciate yourself as you are, to notice your good intentions and accomplishments, and to care for yourself as tenderly as you would for someone else that you love. Cultivate the attitude of feeling like there is all the time in the world. You can tell that you are being nurtured when you are relaxed and unhurried and have a sense that life, even with its pain and disappointments, is basically worth living.

WITH OTHER PEOPLE.

Like most women, I was raised to tend to the needs of others to the exclusion of my own. I found it difficult to put myself in social situations and form personal relationships that would nurture *me*—even after I was diagnosed with arthritis and became convinced that this would help me to function and live a "normal" life again. A therapist even suggested that it was a matter of *life and death* for me to find nurturing connections, since my disease is systemic and crippling. Her dramatic declaration increased my motivation to forge such connections. I began by observing the impact that being with other people had on my pain and energy level. After months of such observation, I started to understand what kinds of social relationships actually nurture me. I tend to want to feel needed by others. I also need to be acknowledged and admired by others. After I understood what kinds of relationships met my needs, I began to structure my life so that these kinds of relationships were possible.

Social relationships. I was surprised to discover that social situations were more complicated than I had originally supposed. I always automatically attended obligatory social functions and usually had a good time. Then I went home and went about my own life. I rarely initiated social engagements myself, such as asking friends to accompany me to some musical or theatrical event. Usually other people called me, and I went if I had no strong feelings against going. The new revelation was that in social situations that were set up by others, I wasn't always nurtured. Large groups of people and superficial chatter tend to drain my energy rather than raise it. Now I seldom go to large parties (four or more people) unless I expect to receive warm attention and to be stimulated by the conversation. If for some reason—maybe I'm in an adventurous mood or I want to meet a particular guest of honor—I choose to go to a party where most of the people will be unknown and therefore indifferent to me, I always wear or carry something that will provoke curious inquiry, and thus my rapacious need for attention will be met.

Socially I am nurtured when in the company of energetic, amiable people who are lively enough to focus their attention on subjects of mutual interest and to partake in activities that I enjoy immensely. I love to bicycle with friends, but *not* with friends who chatter about real estate prices while we are cruising through breathtaking scenery.

While I was gathering information about my social needs, I discovered that the most reliable gauge of whether I am being nurtured in company is whether my energy is increased or decreased in a social situation. If I am in the company of one other person and that person is covertly manipulating me in some way—usually by forcing me into some kind of role that does not acknowledge my individuality, such as being a sounding board for his or her emotional grievances—I am not being nurtured. I am being put upon, and I can feel my energy begin to drain slowly out of my body if I tolerate this imposition. I've learned to decline the invitations of people whose expectations of me feel very narrow or static, or who demand that I fulfill a role that is not satisfying to me.

I never go out with friends I am angry with unless we are going to discuss the reasons for my anger. You are *not* being nurtured if you feel restless, dissatisfied, anxious about having fulfilled your obligations, or manipulated by other people. A good criterion for companionship is to choose friends whose needs are being met at the same time your needs are being met; what you do together is mutually satisfying.

When friends and loved ones give me gifts, I note internally the habitual feelings of embarrassment such tribute evokes. Then I let these feelings fade and allow myself to bask in the affection that prompted such a gesture. I have observed that people often don't allow themselves to feel the emotional bounty that may be available to them, to reap the emotional rewards of being highly regarded by the important people in their life. We often take our friends and loved ones and their esteem for granted. Hugs and words of appreciation are important to us biochemically. *Allow yourself to feel nurtured by those who love you.*

I married after I got arthritis, not before. Feeling independent had been more important to me than being intimate with another person; I finally traded some of my independence for nurturing.

Family relationships. It is often difficult to begin to face a disability or a great deal of pain within a family situation because you may be abandoning your usual role in your family. This role change may provoke feelings of guilt and failure. (Of course, it is probably more difficult to face disability *without* the support of an understanding and loving family.) Families may fail to be supportive for various reasons.

- Outside stresses and intrafamilial demands are already so great that the family cannot absorb another crisis.
- The arthritic person served the family by always being in the supportive role for other family members. The other members not only don't know how to reverse roles and offer support themselves, but don't even know how to continue functioning without the stricken one's support. This may be true of children who have never been asked to assume any responsibility within the family.
- The arthritic person only knows how to obtain support by manipulating and bullying other family members.

A family counselor may be needed to help you discover the reasons familial support is not forthcoming and to gradually change the situation—if remaining within the family is to be part of your healing rather than a distraction to healing. Just as a loving family can contribute tremendously to a healing atmosphere by providing the chronically ill person with a stable emotional base, a resentful, conflicted family can sabotage the healing process by fostering strife and tension. Even if there is no open confrontation, a tense atmosphere full of unspoken anger can be more corrosive than open hostility.

Family members may feel resentment without knowing it, without consciously intending any malice toward the sick person. They may feel disoriented at first; a family member whose support they have counted on has withdrawn into his or her own problems. There is no longer as much attention to go around as there once was. A spouse may end up shouldering more responsibility than he or she can handle. A child may feel abandoned in some subtle way that is not acknowledged or explained by the adults. Family members may feel guilty about their resentment. Or their wish to preserve an atmosphere of normalcy may be so strong that they remain unconscious of these negative feelings.

It is very important to the healing process and for all members of the family that these feelings are allowed to be acknowledged without blame. It is natural to feel them.

A child must understand that he or she is not the cause of the parent's or sibling's chronic illness. Children are extremely egocentric and attribute all world events to their own feelings and behavior. They may think that some "naughtiness" or "bad thought" caused or is aggravating the illness of their parent or sibling. Children should receive as much information as possible in such situations. They should be informed about the extent of the disability, care and prognosis, and their own roles within the household. Clearly explaining such details is very important in warding off guilt and anxiety.

Whenever I was in a very bad mood because of pain, I passed this information to my son early in the day. Then he and I both knew that I could complain and he could protest. I felt relief when I, in a very irritable state of mind, scolded him, and he replied, equally irritably, "Just because you feel bad doesn't mean you have to make other people feel bad." I tried to give him permission to express himself, and he did. Today I feel gratitude and pride that my son was able to distinguish between my arthritis and my essential being, my humanity.

Sexual relationships. Because arthritis varies so much from day to day, there will be some days when you feel too weak and uncomfortable to engage in sexual relations. Your sexual partner is especially vulnerable to feelings of humiliation and rejection if you do not tell him or her why you don't want sex on these occasions. You must take the initiative and strive to be very clear and considerate of your nonarthritic mate. You should not have sex when you don't feel up to it—although in my experience sex does wonders for mild stiffness. Remember, the onus is on you to make it clear to your mate if you don't want sex because your arthritis is acting up.

I can deal with this issue when my body hurts me enough to preclude any sexual activity—at least then the situation is clear-cut. My problem is that sometimes even when I am functional, I just don't want to *feel* my body. For a long time, whenever my husband stroked me affectionately, I immediately felt despair. It took me a while to realize that what I was feeling was the deep sadness residing in my body, the grief over the fading of its youthful vigor into the clumsy stiffness of arthritis. What I eventually learned to do was to take refuge from the despair in my husband's loving arms.

For a period of months, sex was very difficult for me. I had very little energy; I was completely wrapped up in my efforts toward self-sufficiency, and my body ached a great deal. Getting to the bathroom and brushing my teeth was an accomplishment; I certainly didn't feel like exerting myself sexually. Just the heat and weight of my husband's body were onerous. He couldn't help being angry, if not directly at me, then angry in general. I often wondered if he would leave me and find someone else. Sometimes I thought I should have the grace to leave first so that he could find a suitable mate without the guilt of leaving his crippled wife. I tried not to belabor these thoughts, but they were the kind that crept into my head at three o'clock in the morning.

What saved us (and me) was that we really were determined to make our relationship work on every level. We began to formalize our attempts at solving these problems. Every morning when we woke up, he asked how I felt. Every morning I told him truthfully: "I feel better," "I feel just awful," or "I feel pretty good." No matter how I felt, this ritual seemed to give me permission to feel that way. Now I was neither concealing my pain nor feeling I was imposing it on my husband.

Every evening when my husband and I saw each other again after the day's separation, he would again inquire how I felt. If I said I felt good, he knew he could hold me and caress me without an explicit invitation. Where this led was up to the two of us. I tried to be clear and accurate about my availability. Still, in general, we were not having sex as often as he desired.

We finally hit on a solution. Once a month we devoted a weekend to sex and love. Both of us cleared our calendars and either stayed home or went to a bed-and-breakfast for the weekend. There I dressed in clothes that made me feel beautiful and desirable rather than grumpy and arthritic. We paced our activities according to my energy level: maybe biking or swimming, maybe a movie or dinner out, maybe just lying in bed and alternately resting and making love for two whole days. I can't adequately convey my deep pleasure in resolving to make this work, nor my great love for and gratitude to my husband for being such a resourceful, loving, and sexual man.

Dietary Considerations

The classic arthritis diet is well-known and available from a variety of sources, including doctors' offices and health food stores. Basically, this diet consists of fresh fruit and vegetables (with exceptions noted below) and a protein source such as fish, chicken, or whole grains. Moderate consumption is recommended. Almost all arthritis diets prohibit dairy foods, meat, sugar, alcohol, salt, spicy foods, and fat. Some preclude fish, chicken, wheat, nightshades (potatoes and tomatoes), and citrus.

Some people with arthritis are helped dramatically by monitoring their diets, whereas others get no results. There is great variation among arthritics in symptoms, prognosis, and course of the disease, so of course there are huge variations in the effectiveness of any diet or supplement to control the symptoms. For some of my clients, an arthritis diet has proved to be the most effective treatment they have tried; for most of them, it has been somewhat helpful in that it decreases pain and stiffness without eliminating them. Others have found that although no particular diet is very effective, some foods (usually alcohol or sweets) greatly aggravate symptoms.

I feel I must say a few things about restrictive diets in general. Basically, I don't think going on a rigid, self-denying regimen is helpful for anyone with arthritis. This just tends to reinforce the rigid, highly unpleasant situation that already exists. It is important to break through the restrictions of arthritis, to have a positive sense of self-nourishment and of *bounty*. Therefore, anyone embarking on a diet for his or her health ought to be flexible with regard to food choices. (For more on this topic see chapter 6.)

The reason a certain diet will ease your arthritis is not that going on it makes you a virtuous person who deserves the relief. The diet eases the symptoms of arthritis because one of those symptoms is your body's inability to digest foods thoroughly and carry away waste materials (what's left after your body has used the portion of your food it's broken down for nutrients). If you have a systemic disease, the disease process damages the red blood cells that carry oxygen (necessary for the digestion of food) and nutrients to all body cells and carry away waste products. If you have degenerative arthritis, your tissues are prone to swelling for climatic (and possibly physiological) reasons, and digestion and waste removal are impaired. So if you eat foods in reasonable quantities that are relatively easy to digest (fruits and vegetables), if you don't clog up your system with excess wastes (sweets, alcohol, fats), and if you facilitate digestion by drinking lots of water, you are minimizing the load you are putting onto a system that is already burdened by disease.

Sometimes your symptoms are greater, sometimes less, depending on how your system is functioning at the moment. You may deduce that a food that often bothers you doesn't always. When you are feeling great, your joints are free from soreness, and your energy is high, you can indulge in a food that you don't ordinarily dare eat. By becoming familiar with your body's ability to process toxins, you can learn to rely on your own personal judgment about what to eat, when, and how much on any particular occasion while maintaining your body's comfort level. Often for weeks or months at a time, I can eat whatever I like. But when I start feeling some general malaise or particularly sore, I realize that it's time to watch the quantity of food that I eat and shift to a higher proportion of vegetables to grains. It is also necessary for me to eliminate sugar, alcohol, and meat altogether for the duration of my flare-up.

Movement that Heals

Movement has a tremendously beneficial effect on the various systems of the body, including the immune system. Specifically, I refer to the kind of movement that relaxes and soothes the musculature and organic systems of the body and that also stimulates the nervous system and expands the possibilities for new patterning in the brain. Healing movements relieve stress and muscle fatigue and lead to better, less effortful movement in general. They create a sense of the body's axis, or center. If we feel subtly off-center when we move, we create discombobulating tension in our bodies. We must come back to rest in the center of our body for that tension to fall away. Healing movement also increases the use of a number of muscles, particularly small muscles, in the body so that we don't repeatedly strain the same large muscles while allowing major portions of our bodies to remain unused and flaccid. When you move, all your bones should be supported by a network of muscles that complement each other and share between them the effort of your exertion. When we overuse large muscles by performing the same routine motions over and over again, we fail to develop small, very specific muscles. As a result, our movements are clumsy, unbalanced.

Movement should also enhance joint mobility and pain-free function. Instead of compressing and contracting joints by forcing movement in such a way that joints are damaged, we can use movement to extend our head, arms, and legs when we move. *Because we must move anyway in our daily activities, we might as well learn to move in ways that enhance our well-being rather than threaten it.*

Healing movement is movement that follows the rhythm set by our breathing. Many people hold their breath when they concentrate or move so that movement of some muscles must come into conflict with others. The whole body expands and relaxes when movement is in sync with breathing. Our bodies were created to move and breathe. Most of us need to activate dormant muscles and liberate our breathing in order to feel more alive.

The same movement can be beneficial at one point in your healing but counterproductive at another point. It depends on whether that movement promotes or detracts from the expansion of your body at a given moment. For a person with arthritis, taking a walk on a particular day may not be a good idea, even though it was helpful the day before. If the joints are so constricted and the body is so tight that the body contracts rather than expands as the person walks, walking will not be a beneficial exercise for that individual.

A person may have very strong postural muscles and thus look capable of walking for exercise, when in fact only a few muscles are very strong and most of them are very weak; therefore, the strong muscles are continually strained while the person is walking. So nothing is gained or changed; the person's body persists in its straining, weakening patterns, and the exercise becomes degenerative rather than regenerative.

The person must alter the pattern of movement sufficiently to exercise new muscles and to stimulate new patterns in the brain so that he or she has a different conception of the body's capabilities. Movement that generates new patterns is a healing exercise; just moving in the same old stiff way is not.

The problem with exercise "routines" that require repetition of the same motion is that the body gets used to that motion and becomes self-limited by moving repeatedly in the same way, using the same muscles and continuing to neglect others. If you wish to change a routine motion into a healing one, you can ask yourself: What does this movement feel like? What part of my body is moving? What part is not moving? What part is relaxed? What does my breathing feel like? Does it feel good to do this motion? What could I add to expand this motion, to increase my mobility while doing it? Changing a routine motion to a healing, inspiring one involves taking a new attitude toward the motion.

For instance, if you do leg lifts to strengthen your quadriceps (front thigh muscles) and have done that exercise for months or even years, you may do it automatically by now, hardly noticing what it feels like to do it. In fact, it may have been some time since you actually noticed any improvement in the strength of your thighs, but you continue to do the same exercise the same way because you fear losing the strength you once gained if you stop doing it.

To increase the effectiveness of your leg lifts, energize your exercise sessions, and generally expand your conception of move-

ment in your hip and upper leg, ask yourself: What lifts my leg when I raise it? What other muscles besides my quadriceps are helping to lift my leg? Does my back help? Does my abdomen help? Can I lift my leg with my thigh alone? Is my breathing regular? Is my upper body totally independent of the movement of my leg lifting? These questions not only stimulate your awareness of your body (and therefore your interest in exercising it) but will eventually lead to much more efficient strengthening of your quadriceps because you will eventually learn to isolate your quadriceps muscles from the rest of your body and therefore to use *only* your quadriceps muscles to do your leg lifts. This will strengthen your leg much faster than if you unconsciously help your quadriceps by using your abdomen and back muscles.

Anytime you exercise specifically to help your body, you should become mobile in your other activities as a result. If you don't, you haven't gained anything. Ideally, every time you move at all, you should move in such a way that your mobility is promoted. When you move a pot from the stove to the table, or walk to the store, you have an opportunity to work on your long-term healing. If you have a degenerative disease, all your movements not only should perform a necessary function but should instruct your brain in further mobility. Are your old patterns determining the way you do your arthritis exercises? It is much more helpful for you if you do your exercises in such a way that your habits of movement are challenged. You will know that is happening if you walk differently after your exercises. Your exercise sessions should inspire healing instead of merely reinforcing old habit patterns in your body that got you into trouble in the first place.

Breath's Healing Power

We all know that breathing enables the body to obtain oxygen to carry out its functions. Some of us also realize that one of the main functions of blood is to carry oxygen and nourishment to all parts of the body. But beyond this general knowledge, most of us don't think too much about breathing or oxygen. Before you were diagnosed with arthritis, the odds are that you rarely noticed the expansion and contractions of your diaphragm as you breathed and how profoundly (albeit unconsciously) this indicated that all was right with the world.

Now that you have arthritis, however, you may have a new appreciation and respect for the breathing process and for the role that oxygen plays in the body. Your food is broken down into simpler and simpler sugars only in the presence of oxygen. If you lack oxygen because your lung capacity is reduced, your food is not broken down com-

pletely. This means that the food that could have contributed further to your nutrition becomes instead another undigested waste product in your blood. It then adds to the congestion in your system caused by your disease. So just on this biochemical level alone, it is vital to learn to breathe fully and regularly.

If your movements have become somewhat or very restricted because of arthritis and you feel your body is clumsy, jerky, and unbalanced, you need to become conscious of your breathing to reestablish a sense of balance and rhythmic motion. By focusing on your breathing as you walk, for instance, you can feel your body parts begin to become independent of each other as your breath goes in and out. You may unconsciously hold your shoulders up around your ears. Every time you exhale, your shoulders have the chance to relax. If you can feel your breath leave your body, your shoulders can ease down, let go, move. This is much more effective in relieving shoulder pain than forcing the shoulders down with the shoulder muscles. You will feel much more comfortable if your shoulders fall down on your out-breath than if you push them down with your determination.

The loosening effect of focusing on breathing during movement is tremendous. Your extremities (your head, arms, and legs) seem to move out into space, away from your torso, as you move. You become aware of your torso as the locus of all basic functions, as your head, arms, and legs perform your activities. Your head moves out of your torso toward the sky; your arms pull out of your shoulders (stretching the joints as they extend) to manipulate things; your legs swing out of your hips to place your feet on the ground. Feeling your extremities "fall off" your torso gives you a wonderful sense of unfettered movement.

To bring an awareness of your breathing into your daily life, try breathing deeply every hour on the hour, but don't be hard on yourself when you forget to do this for several hours in a row. Just keep trying to do it day after day until it is part of your consciousness.

I also recommend that you take some time, whether it is a day or even an hour, to assess your breathing as an indicator of how comfortable and relaxed you are feeling. Do only those activities and see only those people that you associate with deep and relaxed breathing; avoid those activities and people that you associate with shallow and restricted breathing. You will discover a great deal about the way you have been spending your time and energy, certainly enough to decide whether you wish to continue spending them that way.

Exercises

The following exercises will help you increase your lung capacity along with your awareness of the whole breathing process. They should all be done while lying on your back.

HOLDING BREATH IN AND LETTING IT OUT. Take a deep breath and hold it in to a count of ten, then let it out. When all your breath has been exhaled, count to eight before you breathe in again. Repeat, counting to progressively larger numbers (fifteen, twelve; twenty, fifteen; twenty-five, twenty) as your capacity for air increases. This exercise will help you learn to inhale and exhale thoroughly, which is especially helpful if you have asthma.

FEELING THE BREATH MOVE THE ABDOMEN. Breathe deeply. Place your hands on the sides of your abdomen so you can feel your abdomen expand and shrink as your breath goes in and out. This exercise gives you a sense of how your breath moves the muscles of your body. You can feel movement so definite that it displaces your hands as you breathe in and out.

WAVE BREATHING. Breathe normally, allowing your breath to deepen naturally as you relax. When you feel relaxed, begin to suck in your stomach with your stomach muscles and puff out your chest with your chest muscles at the same time that you breathe in and out. Collapse your chest and push out your stomach. Suck in your stomach and puff out your chest again; then collapse your chest and push out your stomach, over and over again, creating a wave motion as you go back and forth between your chest and your stomach. Continue until you feel looser through your whole torso, front and back.

BELLY STRENGTHENER. Breathe normally until you feel relaxed. Then take a deep breath and hold it in. Use your abdominal muscles first to push your belly out as far as you can and then to suck your belly in as far as you can—all while still holding your breath. Continue to move your belly in and out while you hold your breath. Then, when you need to exhale, breathe out and repeat the movement—moving your belly up and down with your abdominal muscles—without breathing in again until absolutely necessary. After inhaling, repeat the movement once more. Continue in this fashion until you need a rest. Try doing this exercise for five minutes at a time, including rest periods. In a few weeks you probably will be able to do the exercise for the whole five minutes without rest periods. If you can't, don't worry about it. This exercise is very good for you. It is more effective than sit-ups in strengthening your abdominal muscles.

CHEST STRENGTHENER. Follow the instructions for the above exercise using your chest to move your breastbone up and down (as

you used your abdominal muscles to move your belly in and out).

THROAT MUSCLE STRENGTHENER. Follow the instructions for the belly strengthener using your throat muscles to move your clavicle bones, just below your throat, up and down.

SOUNDING. Take a deep breath, then let it out while making a humming sound at the back of your throat. Repeat with every outbreath, only practice moving the humming sound deeper and deeper down the front of your body to your abdomen. Feel the vibration of your sound in your bones.

After you get the hang of this, try other sounds as well: moaning, all the vowels—*a, e, i, o, u*—and "hoo" sounds like the wind. Notice where these different sounds resonate; some will resonate in your chest, some up in your head. Sounding is especially helpful if you are feeling very constricted in your chest and belly, as if you don't have enough room in your upper body to breathe. The vibration in your chest produced by sounding may introduce a sense of spaciousness that leads to deeper, easier breathing.

Some people find breathing exercises difficult to do because they are more subtle than moving external muscles, like those in your arms or legs, and require more of your attention, especially at first. You may have become impatient at times while trying to find the internal muscles that differentiate movements between your chest and stomach. It is worth persisting, however, because breath is at the heart of living with your body as it is in any given moment. If you can develop the presence to follow your breath as it goes in and goes out for a period of time, you will be cultivating your ability to become immersed in the mundane events of your everyday life—the breeze against your cheek as you step outside, the comforting sensation of your clothes against your skin as you move—and your reward will be a life so infinitely rich with detail that pain cannot commandeer your attention.

Chapter 4

How to Work on Joints

People with arthritis need to maintain a healthy immune system, as discussed in chapter 3, but they also must work locally on arthritic joints to prevent or reverse damage. If the joint is inflamed, nutrients are not being carried to the cartilage and bone, and waste materials are not being carried out by the bloodstream. When the body does not function efficiently enough to remove waste materials from the joints, it is necessary to cleanse the joints mechanically to prevent further deterioration. Anti-inflammatory drugs and painkillers are routinely used for this purpose. A more wholesome alternative may be movement and massage. The kind of movements that are most effective in reducing inflammation, relaxing contracted tissue, and restoring balance to arthritic joints are gentle, subtle, and very specific movements that directly affect the area.

A Warning Against Doing Vigorous Exercise Before You Are Loose

Vigorous exercises like jogging or playing tennis use large muscle groups, and although they increase general circulation throughout the body, they do not necessarily increase the efficiency of local circulation in a specific area or joint, especially if that area is habitually tight because of muscle tension or pain. If some parts of the body are held rigidly during strenuous activity, local joints are not receiving the blood supply they need for oxygen and waste management. It is a common notion that exercises must be strenuous or tiring to be effective, but actually the reverse is true. If you strain and overuse the same areas of your body repeatedly, while neglecting to increase the circulation and mobility of stiff parts, you are harming rather than healing yourself.

Many exercise programs prescribed for arthritis make the mistake of trying to strengthen weak muscles before loosening the tight, stiff joints between them. Exercises that require too much effort stress tight, painful joints. The problem may be not the type of strengthening exercises themselves but the fact that the stiff joints have not been prepared by sufficient loosening to bear such a burden. The same strengthening exercises are fine *after* you have loosened up your joints with smaller, more precise, and relaxing motions. You should not attempt to stretch or strengthen muscle tissue around a joint before that joint is loose, that is, before it is relatively pain-free and able to at least approximate its original range of motion. Only a joint that moves freely in all directions, that is able to rotate in a fluid, circular motion, not an angular, jerky one, is ready to meet the demands of leg lifts and stretches.

Whenever you have pain during your exercise session, do not ignore it or continue with the movements! Stop and address your discomfort. It is discouraging and potentially damaging to work against your pain. When you are in pain, you need to ease the joints that hurt—discover the movements that re-lease you, not challenge you. (For a discussion of how to do this, see pages 10–20.)

The Advantages of Gentle Movement

There is a great deal of wisdom in being willing to start at the very beginning: to steadily unlock your joints and muscles with gentle, slow movements that loosen your body and increase its capacity to move. After the joints in your body or in a specific area of your body have relaxed, expanded, and recovered some mobility, you can increase that mobility by going on to stretching the muscles, tendons, and ligaments around those joints and then strengthening the muscles around them. A fully mobile joint will receive nutrients from the blood, and it will give up its waste products into the bloodstream as well. Even if cartilage has been damaged already, it is possible to restore a great deal of flexibility and strength to the damaged joint if you are patient enough to work with it gently until it is no longer very sore. Then, when you're free of pain, you can do the kind of demanding exercise that builds strength. Strong muscles cushion the pressure of joint use. Flexible tendons and ligaments protect the stability or balance of the joint. It is important to maintain or restore these conditions. In this way you can work on eliminating any restriction you have, even if you have had it for a long time.

Spending an hour on your bed or the floor gently moving several small parts of the body at the same time that you breathe deeply is dramatically and profoundly healing because it relaxes the muscles, stimulates the brain, flushes the joints, and cleans the blood, even though you are not even winded at the end. Of course, you must do other exercises to maintain heart-lung fitness; however, if you relax your whole body and loosen specific joints first, your aerobic exercise will truly help you rather than merely tire and strain you. There are several advantages to small, gentle movements:

• *The small loosening movements are very stimulating to the nervous system because they introduce the idea of "no limitation" during movements to people who have become accustomed to feeling restriction in their movements.* These movements are so small and precise that even very stiff people feel "loose" doing them. The brain perceives space and flow where there was limitation before. Thus, your exercise session inspires you instead of merely reinforcing old habit patterns of stress and strain while moving. It is wonderful to feel loose, to move well within your range and comfort; this new feeling of expanding boundaries carries over into how you approach everyday tasks. You'll be able to stretch with pleasure when you reach for a cup on the shelf, or to feel your legs stretch out from your hips when you walk.

• *Small movements are easily tracked by your brain.* You feel more of what is happening when you make small movements slowly and precisely, rather than vigorously move a large area of your body. Whenever you pay attention to what your body feels when you move, your brain can use that information to solve whatever difficulty you are having. If you try many small movements in lying, sitting, and standing positions, your brain gets a great deal of information about what exactly influences the comfort of your joints.

• *Small movements increase the network of muscles supporting moving bones.* Developing muscles, particularly small muscles, provides "definition" to your body and improves its grace and function. This is important so that you do not repeatedly strain the same large muscles over and over again in your activity. The fewer the muscles, the grosser the movement; one becomes limited to several large movements in a few directions with no variation. The support of small muscles allows small, subtle movements that keep the body supple and protect all muscles and bones from the impact of vigorous movement.

• *Small movements promote relaxation and enjoyment.* Various body therapies developed in the last twenty years rely on small, gentle movements to provide the kind of soothing, comforting stimulation that people in pain require. You are more likely to stick with a daily exercise period when it feels good to move than when you dread returning to an uncomfortable routine.

Most of the movements suggested in this book are rotations of one part of the body around another part. That is because rotational movements are full, multidirectional movements that gently stretch all the muscles and connective tissue around each joint, unlike many exercises that require repetitive movement in only one direction (e.g., handball, pedaling an exercycle, conventional leg lifts). Repetitive movements activate only a few muscles and nerves—some muscles are stretched or strengthened while others are neglected, leading to imbalance in the joint. Multidirectional movements flood your brain with information about your joints, all of them, in every possible way. Whenever you're in pain, you should have "on file" in your brain a multitude of strategies for easing the part that hurts or all of your body. You know from past experience which kinds of movements will be the most likely to provide relief. The more precise and varied the movements you experience, the greater your storehouse of movements to make pain-free functioning possible.

Passive Movement: An Important Technique

One kind of very pleasant passive movement is when someone else moves a part of your body. You lie there, giving over your leg or arm to someone who moves you while you experience the sensation of movement. We enjoy this type of activity because it feels so good to relinquish to someone else the effort movement ordinarily requires. No weight on our joints, no pull on our muscles, no place to move ourselves to. We have only the sweet sensation of movement. Even if your joints are usually very painful with movement, they often can be moved without any pain if someone else does the moving. This should tell you there may be something about the way you move that is hurting your joints.

For most of us, it isn't feasible to have someone else move us every time we want relief. The good news is that you can do this for yourself. You can have one part of your body moved passively by another part of your body so that the part that is moved is eased, soothed, and relaxed. For instance, if your hips hurt, your bent knees moving gently together from side to side can relax and soothe your hips. If your shoulders hurt, you can reach over with one hand to move the opposite shoulder gently into a more comfortable position. If your neck hurts, moving the very top of your head in a small circular motion will relax your neck muscles. The boon of passive movement is that you can ease most pains all by yourself.

Massage and Movement

I highly recommend that you massage joints before, during, and after the movements discussed in this book. (The same advice applies to all vigorous activities.) If you feel some discomfort doing any of the movements described here, try massaging the problem area while you do the movement. When I first began working on my own damaged joints, some of the more painful ones were extremely resistant to movement. If I moved them even a little more than they were accustomed to being moved, they would flare up in great pain. Massage is very important when you begin to penetrate your stiffness. You must soothe and comfort stressed joints by massaging them in order to move them more. Not only will massage make you feel better—no small thing in itself—but it will reduce the inflammation, or irritation, which new movement may have provoked. It is necessary to be very patient with joints that have not moved much in recent times. You need to apply a little bit of movement, a lot of massage, a little bit more movement, a lot more massage, until the joint stops swelling in reaction to the movement, and its range of motion is thereby increased.

Stretching and Strengthening

Severely damaged joints may take a great deal of tiny, passive moving (your manually rotating your ankle or knee with your hand, for instance) and massage before they begin to move more easily and less painfully on their own. During this initial period it is important to be patient, to continue to massage

and passively move the joint until it has clearly improved before attempting to stretch or strengthen it. You will know that stretching is appropriate when stretching makes your joint feel better, not worse. Sometimes if my shoulders are mildly achy (but still fully functioning and able to bear the weight of my arms), stretching my arms out will make the pain disappear altogether. But if my shoulders are very stiff and acutely painful, stretching them only makes me catch my breath with pain. In that case, I stop immediately and return to very simple, gentle loosening movements. (The various loosening movements are included in chapter 10.)

After stretching a joint makes it feel vital and warm, you can safely begin to do strengthening exercises with it. In chapter 10 I will list strengthening exercises for each joint, but of course conventional sports activities such as biking, swimming, or playing ball are all strengthening activities for some parts of the body. It is good to notice which muscles are affected by the play you do and to supplement that activity with exercise that works other areas of your body so that all your large muscles are worked over a week's time.

Setting Aside an Exercise Time

The way people usually exercise in our culture—counting ten repetitions to the left, then ten to the right—tends to make movements mechanical and boring. It interferes with one's ability to concentrate on and feel the sensations of the movements. I suggest that you set aside a certain amount of time to exercise, say a half hour or an hour, or longer if you come to enjoy doing the movements. Don't count repetitions; instead set a timer to inform you when the period is over. That enables you to concentrate on feeling your bodily sensations rather than trying to cram as many motions into the exercise session as possible. You can start with where you hurt or where you feel restriction and perform the movements that ease your pain or expand your ability to move.

One set of movements often arouses a desire in your body to do another related, but different, set of movements that move slightly different muscles. As you relieve one area, another part of you comes to your attention. In this way you work on different parts of your body in various ways until your time is up. If you are very restricted in one or two areas, you may prefer to do just a few movements in only one area the whole time. Either way, you will be meeting the unique needs of your own situation. This makes for an extremely effective and efficient exercise session.

Exercise Strategy

An important way to approach exercise is to do exercises without having any goal in mind. It may seem difficult for someone with a disability to suspend the thought of working toward eliminating or ameliorating that disability, but it is very relaxing, and therefore healing, to have some time each day when the body is not under the stress of working toward a goal. Even healing as a goal can become oppressive—it's like frantically trying to "relax."

A more productive state of mind for exercising is that of self-awareness. The mind focuses on physical or emotional sensations and feelings. It imposes no demands. You do what it feels good to do. You contact the "boundlessness" in yourself. Healing arises from this state of mind.

When I am feeling well and my exercise sessions are not devoted to soothing and loosening my painful body, I enjoy starting the sessions with a challenging movement like standing, then bending to touch my toes. I monitor my restrictions, noticing, let's say, a tightness in my hamstrings, inflexibility of my lower spine, and stiffness in my left ankle. Then I work on each restriction in turn.

Standing in front of a table, I raise one leg onto a pillow on the table; then, breathing deeply and slowly, I stretch toward the toes of the elevated leg. Then I alternate legs. I am very careful not to stretch farther than each breath allows so that I am not tearing the muscle fiber in my hamstrings. After I am able to stretch farther toward my toes than I could when I started alternating my legs to

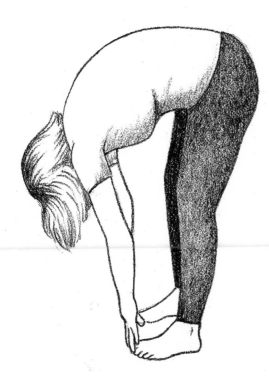

foot onto the seat, knee bent. I lean forward and begin to rotate my left leg at the knee. This moves my ankle at every angle, further releasing the lower leg muscles and increasing the angle of the flex as I rotate. I continue this rotation until my ankle moves easily in every direction: forward and back, left and right.

I return to toe touching. This time not only my fingers but also my hands touch the floor. My ankle is loose, my spine is loose, my hamstrings are loose. By identifying and working on the various restrictions that prevented me from touching my toes, I have used my exercise session to accomplish that position. I end my session not only looser but triumphant!

Working on your body without a goal doesn't mean you can't have long-term goals for your body. You may want to be able to climb the stairs without leaning on the railing. Or to play golf again. These are goals to try out occasionally, but they cannot dominate your thinking during your exercise session without compromising your ability to feel what the capacity of your body is *right now* and to work on reducing your restrictions.

When I first began to walk again after spending so much time in bed with arthritis, I noticed that my legs never straightened all the way at the knee. I was embarrassed to wear short skirts because it was obvious in the mirror that my knees were bent even

the table, I go back to the original standing exercise and try touching my toes again. I can go farther.

Now it's time to work on my lower spine. I lie on my back, and with my knees pulled up against my chest and held with my arms, I rock my pelvis forward and back, gently stretching the muscles in my lower spine. After I feel relaxed and loose in my lower back, however long it takes, I get up again and try to touch my toes. I feel my upper body shift toward the floor as my lower spine releases it. It is tremendously satisfying and physically pleasant to feel that shift. Now the remaining restriction I feel is in my left ankle.

Standing in front of a chair, I lift my left

though I stood as straight as I could. I decided I wanted straight legs and would get them.

First I identified the restriction. I could feel that when I attempted to straighten my knees, there was a great deal of crunching and some sharp pain deep inside as though the bones of my femur and tibia (upper and lower leg) were too close to each other to allow the knee to straighten. I realized that since I was probably dealing with the position of the bones as well as the inflexibility of connective tissue, it would take a long time to fix this problem. But given normal life expectancy, I had a long time. I was thirty-eight years old.

Next I decided on a tentative strategy. It seemed to me I needed stronger quadriceps muscles (those in the front of the thigh), looser hamstring muscles (those in the back of the thigh), and well-balanced adductors (those inside the thigh). Plus, judging from the crunching sound that accompanied any attempt to straighten my knees, I needed more room in the joint for the bones to move around each other. My X rays showed damaged cartilage, so I wouldn't get much help there. I would have to rely on strong and flexible muscles, tendons, and ligaments.

After deciding which movements would stretch and strengthen all my thigh muscles and which would loosen the knee joint (that is, tell my brain there was enough space in the knee to move easily), I devoted ten min-utes a day to those exercises. I began by gently rotating my lower legs around my knees for a few minutes while I sat in a chair until my knees felt warm and loose. Then I lay down on my back and put one leg into the air as straight as I could without pain or the crunching sound. I moved the leg from side to side, to the outside of my body, then across it, until it moved to both sides easily. Then I put it down and did the same with the other leg. Finally, I sat up and massaged each knee in turn for a minute or so with oil.

When I first began the leg-in-the-air exercise, I could do it only for a minute or two because it was so difficult. Just putting my leg into the air was all I could do for several weeks. I couldn't move it to either side without touching off uncontrollable and extremely painful spasms that ran up and down from my foot to my hip. My legs were so weak, they couldn't hold their own weight in the air. When they were finally able to stay in the air for as long as I wanted them to, I began to move them slightly from one side to the other, as little as an inch in either direction. This again touched off spasms. These spasms, however, disappeared within a few days, much faster than the original ones had. It took nearly four months to move my legs easily from side to side. But I didn't care how long it took; I was encouraged by any little progress they made, considering how crooked they were.

Once my legs had begun to move easily, I

added another exercise: While sitting on the floor with my legs spread out straight, or nearly straight, in front of me, I inhaled, and then while I exhaled, I stretched toward my toes. I never cared whether or not I was successful in reaching my toes. I knew I would eventually. Meanwhile, the stretch along the backs of my legs and in my lower back felt delicious!

My knees straightened virtually on their own. I did the exercises, and they straightened out. I never pushed them, forced them, or did anything but loosen the knee joint and strengthen the muscles around it. It took about two years. Some people might wonder why I spent two years straightening my knees when I might have had replacement surgery and been off crutches in six months. I preferred straightening my own knees if possible. And not only did my knees straighten, but my hips loosened, my lower back strengthened, and I learned the degree to which I can institute my own healing. I actually lived a full and rich life during the period when I was "incidentally" straightening my knees.

Chapter 5

From the Body's Point of View

Our bodies, sick or well, contain a tremendous amount of information about what it takes to maintain or regain good health. Our health is encapsulated in millions of cell exchanges, chemical reactions, and neurotransmitters that regulate it all. To gain access to that information, scientists have developed the technology to study brain biochemistry. Specialists have begun to concentrate on the neuropeptides and their receptors in order to interpret their influence on emotion and health.

It is possible, however, for us as individuals to access a great deal of information and to influence the course of our health by becoming sensitive to the minutiae of our various bodily processes. When we are suddenly confronted with catastrophic illness, we tend to deny our feelings of pain and devastation or to resign ourselves to our misery. Denial or resignation may be easier than learning to feel, especially if those feelings are painful. But if we are to heal and return to satisfying lives, we must face our feelings; moreover, we must cultivate them and use them to tap the resources of our own body's ability to heal itself.

Because we are more accustomed in our daily lives to the process of thinking (planning, reasoning, judging, creating) than we are to the experience of sensing our bodies, most of us need some instruction on how to receive the information our bodies are always sending us. In this chapter you will learn how to access your body's wisdom.

Why don't we automatically know how to dip into our body's wisdom? Why do we have to learn something that should be instinctual? The answer is that it is indeed instinctual, but most of us have lost our primal connection to our physical beings. We live in a goal-oriented society. We're a nation of doers. We value activities that lead to tangible results, like manufacturing products or designing houses. Many of us experience this emphasis on production as pressure to do as much as possible in as short a time as possible. So as we go about our daily lives, we have a feeling of racing against time.

Even when we intentionally turn our attention to our bodies, as when we do physical exercise, we maintain our goal-orientation. We work out to become stronger, fitter, healthier rather than for any pleasure we feel in the actual doing of such activity. In fact, it is clear from statistics indicating that most of us abandon our workout programs early on that we do not get pleasure from our physical exercise routines.

When we go away on vacation, we have an opportunity to escape the pressure to produce and the feeling of being trapped by time, but for many of us this is such a powerful habit that we continue to pile up the achievements, substituting play activities for work tasks: so many laps in the pool, getting up earlier in order to finish a round of golf by lunch in order to squeeze in a tour before dinner. As a result, many people lead hectic, stress-filled lives, completely estranged from the subtle feelings in their own bodies.

When you lead a goal-oriented life, you pay attention to your ideas, your plans, and your expectations, rather than to your feelings or the sensations of your body. Your body becomes little more than the mobile equipment that gets you across the street and to your appointments—unless you develop some serious physical problem that makes you become more aware of your body.

The following scenario illustrates two different attitudes toward noticing bodily sensation. Let's say you decide to go to the bank. It's a few blocks away, and because of the parking problem, it's easier to walk. What is your mind focusing on as you walk along? Is it the sweet spring air as it brushes your cheek? The sensation of your feet hitting the pavement, causing vibration in your legs and knees? The sensation of your clothes against your skin as your muscles move? The sounds of traffic? The faces of the people you pass? What do you smell? Flowers? The dampness of a recent rain? You may even be aware of your fifth sense if the task of the salty chips or refreshing lemonade you had before your walk lingers in your mouth. These are all internal, timeless, sensate experiences of moving through space. No goal is connected with any of them; your brain is simply organizing the information it receives through your five senses.

Or it may be that your walk to the bank is taken up with thoughts instead of bodily sensations. Perhaps you are thinking of what may happen when you get to the bank. Will you have enough money in your account to cover your withdrawal? Will you have to stand in line? What if you get that teller who annoys you? What are you planning to do after you leave the bank? For some people, these details occupy the mind to the exclusion of any of the actual sensations attendant on walking to the bank. The experiences of the body are not consciously registered. Unfortunately, the ability to register the sensations of the body may atrophy as a muscle does if it is never used.

Why should we develop the ability to feel sensations? Certainly, this adds to the richness of life and the emotional satisfaction to be had from experiencing events on many different levels. And if we do develop some physical difficulty or are interrupted in our function by pain, sensation is where we need to go to find out how to alleviate pain. If you feel pain in your hip when you walk to the bank, which approach do you think will eventually help you: thinking about your bank account, or noticing at what point in your stride the pain comes and goes—and whether experimenting with the way you walk affects it?

Of course, there's nothing wrong with using your intellect. We plan our lives so that we have the resources to enjoy them. We make appointments so that we can conduct business and pleasure with each other. We should be careful, however, not to get "stuck" in one aspect of our rich and multidimensional selves, whatever that aspect is.

Feelings of pain and restriction may focus your attention on the sensations of your body. Stripped of its emotional concomitant, sensation is information—information for your brain about your body. Paying attention to your sensations—for example, under what circumstances you have pain and under what circumstances you don't—can be the basis for your healing in the sense that observations about your difficulty can be used by your brain to formulate a solution to that difficulty. If your hips hurt sometimes but not all the time, you may begin to observe what makes them hurt and what relieves the pain. You try all postures (lying, sitting, and standing) and various movements within those postures, and you begin to get an idea of what exactly influences the comfort of your hips. This is an information-gathering process, your observation of your sensations, and it is crucial to your being able to alleviate that pain.

Using Breath to Feel Your Body

Being aware of the normal rhythms of your breathing is a good way to begin to experience sensation and movement in your body. If you can feel where in your body your breath expands you when you inhale and shrinks you when you exhale, and where it does not expand and shrink you, you can use this awareness of your breath to differentiate one part of your body from another. For example, put your hands on your ribs, right under your chest. You will feel them expand and shrink as you breathe in and out. Move your hand to the edges of this movement, where your breath stops moving your body as you breathe in and out. Perhaps that is your chest. You can feel your ribs being differentiated from your chest every time you breathe. You can feel internally that your ribs are one part of you and your chest is another. Breathe more deeply, and perhaps you can feel your chest muscles expand when you inhale, just as your ribs do. Perhaps now you can distinguish your whole moving midsection from another part that isn't moving with your breath, for instance, your shoulders. Breathe and feel how your midsection is different from your shoulders. You may think, Of course my midsection is different from my shoulders! How obvious! But *feel* the difference. If you are not used to feeling your body and the differences between its different parts, you may be surprised at how subtle these feelings are, how they have to be repeated several times before they attain clarity.

As noted in chapter 3, breathing creates a natural rhythm for your body's movements. If you focus on your breathing as you move, your movements naturally follow that rhythm, and your sense of coordination in-

creases. Stiff, contracted people desperately need to have a sense of grace and coordination as they move. People in pain yearn for some breathing space: around body parts, movements, thoughts, and events. If you focus on your breathing for even a few minutes, you'll glimpse an alternate reality that is compelling in its potential to transform the way you currently endure your pain.

Using Awareness Exercises to Feel Your Body

To acquire the skill of feeling the sensations of our body as we move, most of us need to do specific movements that increase our ability to feel the motion of our body in our everyday activities. The best kind of awareness exercises are those that involve gentle movements, slowly done, so that the brain can easily track the movement we do, and we can therefore feel the sensations that arise in our muscles and joints.

For instance, sit in a chair and put your elbows on the table in front of you. Begin to slowly rotate your hands and forearms around your elbows, both arms at the same time. Your fingertips should lead the motion of your forearms around your elbow; allow your wrists to be loose. Your fingers are active and moving. Feel their effort as you move. Feel the tips of your fingers contact the cool air. Feel your fingers lead the motion

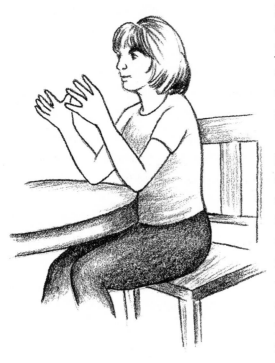

of your forearms around your elbows. Breathe and feel your shoulders, neck, and jaw relax as your arms continue to move.

This is an example of a special exercise that not only relaxes your upper body but is designed to increase your awareness of your upper body sensations as well. The loosening exercises included in chapter 10 are all ideal for developing your ability to track the sensations that different movements produce.

Using Everyday Movements to Feel Your Body

Over the long run, the most effective exercises you will do are the ordinary movements you perform in your everyday life. Why not work on healing your body all day long instead of just one hour of a formal exercise period? After all, you have to move around anyway; you might as well move in a way that enhances rather than compromises your well-being.

In order to begin to move in a way that promotes your ease and healing, you need to start feeling how your everyday movements affect your body. You can assume that when it hurts, you're inadvertently doing something wrong. Arthritis pain is damaging: It impairs blood circulation and squeezes joints with tight, rigidly held muscles. You should do everything you can to avoid it. People in pain often feel the need to do "comforting" movements as they go about their daily tasks. Comforting movements are usually gentle, rhythmic movements that feel like the body is giving itself a little massage. For instance, rotating the hips slowly and soothingly while doing the dishes can be felt as a balm to sore lower body joints. Swinging the arms from side to side can relieve sore shoulders and a stiff upper back. The discomfort of standing in a line at the supermarket can be eased by bending and straightening the knees as you stand in place. Shaking out small, light articles of clothing from the washer can be done loosely and lively enough to make it a treat for stiff elbows and wrists. Once you have developed the habit of tuning in to your body during your everyday activities, you can adapt most of them to healing movements.

What to Do When You Feel Pain

Let's say you move your knee and it hurts. You know from the sensation of pain that you have moved in such a way as to bring the joints of the knee together in a destructive way. In this case, the sensation of pain is your access to the body's wisdom. Your body wants you to stop moving your knee that way. Stop.

Now find a way to move the knee that doesn't hurt. To find a way for your knee to move without hurting, it helps to flood your brain with information about your knee. Does it hurt when you move this way as well? That way? When you do less of the same movement? When you do the same movement in a different direction? Does a different movement make the original movement hurt less when you return to it? The more information your body has about the way you move your knee and all the muscles connected to it, the more possible solutions there are to the original problem of the knee hurting.

In general, the following strategies should prove helpful in lessening or eliminating pain during movement:

• *Stop and pay attention to the pain.* No matter what you're doing and how important you may think it is, you must stop doing it immediately when it causes pain. Give your own comfort level and healing potential a higher priority than the efficient completion of mundane tasks.

• *Do less of the movement that is hurting you.* If you are mixing ingredients in a large bowl, making large circles with your arm to blend the mixture with a spoon, you can make your arm circles smaller. Or you can perform only a portion of the circle, gently folding small amounts of the mixture over itself, so that your arm moves back and forth a small distance along the path of your large motion. You may find that doing a much smaller movement for a little while will enable you to return to the larger movement.

If the pain persists after you return to the larger movement, move your arm on the "frontier" of your pain, the area where movement just begins to be painful but is not quite painful yet. If you move into this area—but stop short of causing real pain—you may expand the area of comfort to include much more of the originally painful movement. In other words, you reduce the amount of territory occupied by pain.

• *Do some movement different from the one that is hurting you.* Often a movement in a different direction or dimension is effective in stretching the joint or releasing the muscle just enough to get the little bit of space in the joint that was needed to eliminate discomfort. If it hurts to move your arm up and down to reach for something on the shelf, try moving it gently across your body a few times, or letting your hand rotate your arm in your shoulder socket as it hangs at your side. Rotation is especially good because it moves the painful area in all directions. Then you can return to the original motion, that is, reaching to the shelf, and see if you have reduced or eliminated the pain.

• *Massage the painful area.* If you have been walking for a while in the park and your ankles start to ache, you can sit down on a bench, lift one of your ankles to your knee, and gently massage the painful, swollen area. Then you can do the same for the other ankle. If you succeed in reducing the swelling by pinching and rubbing the swollen areas, when you get back on your feet, you will feel much better. Or if you suddenly rise

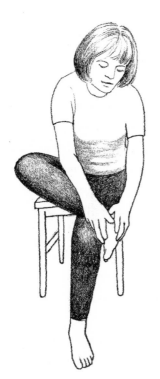

after sitting for a while at your desk, and your hip "catches" and causes you to gasp with pain, you can beat on your hip area gently with your fists and loosen it enough so that you can take steps without discomfort. To administer to yourself in this way, you need some sense that whatever discomfort you feel, you can take care of it yourself.

• *Passively move the painful area with a part more distal to it.* Even if your joints are usually very painful with movement, they often can be moved without pain if someone else does the moving. Use the passive movement technique described in chapter 4 to support one part of your body with another.

In order to become skilled at relieving one part of your body by moving another, more distal part of your body, you need to learn to move different parts of your body independently from each other. If you are relieving a sore hip by moving your leg, you need to feel the muscles in your hip relaxing and gently being moved by the active movement of your leg. It takes practice to develop this skill, as well as concentration on the specific body parts you are attempting to isolate with your movement. If you have difficulty at first determining what part of you is actively moving and what part is being passively moved, ask someone to help you. Your friend can move your leg for you while you concentrate on relaxing your hip. You should notice how it feels for your hip to be passively moved; then you can move your leg so as to duplicate the feeling you had in your hip when your friend was moving your leg. In this way, you can learn how to ease your own pain by moving different parts of your body in relation to each other.

• *Cultivate a state of mind that bypasses pain.* This is a sophisticated strategy, learned and perfected over a long period of time. This state of mind might develop from consistently employing the strategies described above whenever you have pain. Somehow your body/brain learns from how you move and how you breathe what is required to live a relatively pain-free existence. Your body/brain puts together all the information you have been gathering during your daily life movements and your exercise periods and comes up with solutions you could not have consciously managed. This is the potential of the storehouse of information you have gathered by attending to the sensations of your body, those of discomfort, pleasure, and ease. When you can achieve this state of mind every day, or even a few times a week, you are rarely limited in the activities you wish to do by the pangs and fatigue of arthritis.

It is necessary to be consistent in employing these techniques and to remind yourself of what is important in any particular situation: Is it more important that you get the dinner on the stove right this minute, or is it more important to reduce your pain level now? You know that in all cases your health and comfort are more important. Stop and do a few loosening movements and get the dinner on the stove three or four minutes later. When you stop working and address your pain right when it's happening, you not only ease it then, but you are breaking the habit of pain itself. Put your own comfort level and healing potential before the efficient completion of mundane tasks. Stop when it hurts and take the opportunity you have to teach yourself each time how to move without hurting.

Example 1: Taking Your Body's Point of View in the Office

Doing a job from the point of view of your body requires that you develop the mental flexibility to go back and forth between your decision-making mind and the physical sensations of your body. All the actual movements you make—reaching for the phone, settling in your chair—can be done with your mind focused on your bodily feelings. When your job calls for planning, creating, and problem-solving, you must of course focus on abstract concepts, but even so, you can drop into sensation periodically to experience your body.

Here's how to take your body's point of view while doing office work. Start by making the reach across your desk for a pencil into a stretch. Feel your fingers actively, rather than passively, hop from key to key on the word processor. Pick up the phone, and concentrate on the movements of your fingers as they touch the buttons. Notice whether your shoulder is involved in the movements of your fingers, and try to relax your shoulder to the extent that it does not participate. Your fingers are strong enough to push buttons alone. Begin to notice that parts of your body can work while other parts relax. This is essential to reducing pain and increasing stamina as you work.

Feel what supports your body in your chair: Your lower back? Your midback? Your upper back and shoulders? Is there pressure on the back of your neck? Move your spine, upper and lower, until your body settles in your chair. Take care that when you lift your hands and begin to focus your eyes on your work, your spine continues to feel settled and comfortable. As you concentrate on your paperwork, shift your mind back and forth between your work and your body. Check your comfort level, and adjust your posture to relieve pockets of tension in your neck and spine. Move your knees from side to side in the chair to adjust tension in your hips. Rotate your shoulders to relieve tension in your upper spine and neck. Breathe up into your chest to help support your upper spine and neck. Notice how tightly or loosely you hold your pen. Shake your hands out. If you use a word processor or typewriter, notice whether you allow your hands to do your work or whether you tighten your shoulders unnecessarily. Shake your arms out from the shoulders. Notice the muscles in your face and jaw and in your forehead. Rub your cheeks and forehead to relieve tension.

Experiment with your posture. If you work at a terminal, it is very critical to take exercise breaks whenever you can: a few minutes here, even a few seconds there. It is important to change your posture and the focus of your sight as often as possible, at least once an hour. Leave your work periodically to register body sensation mentally. This can be surprisingly revitalizing—or it can be a signal to you that you need to take a real exercise break of three to five minutes or longer. (Refer to chapter 10 for exercises for the upper body.) Take a delicious, high-step-

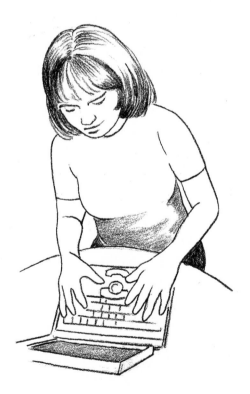

ping walk down to the Xerox machine to copy some work and also to stretch your legs and spine.

Example 2: Doing Physical Work

After having arthritis for several years, I spent a summer on the staff of a resort in Big Sur. Since I was spending most of the day in meetings, I wanted to make certain I had a period of vigorous exercise in the mornings. I requested the job of cabin cleaning, a daily three-hour stint of preparing cabins for new guests. Usually only teenagers were assigned to cabin cleaning because of the prevalent belief that the job required youth and stamina. The duties were clear-cut: replace the sheets, blankets, and bedspreads on every bed, sweep the floor, scour the sink and toilet, empty the trash, and wash the windows and mirrors. The tasks were performed at high speed because anywhere from fifteen to twenty-five cabins needed to be done by lunchtime.

Because there was no conceptual thinking required on this job, I spent the entire work period every day as an exercise session. I did backbends and stretches while changing the bed linens; I twisted my body rhythmically to sweep floors; I stretched every vertebra in my back to scour the toilet; I squeezed the Windex bottle with all five fingers, alternating my hands, to wash the windows. I breathed fully and deeply to set a rhythm for my body movements. After a few weeks of this activity, I was exhilarated and bursting with energy. My posture had improved dramatically from making twenty to forty beds each morning. In contrast, by lunchtime every day almost all of my coworkers (no one over twenty-five and most of them in their teens) would be complaining about their backaches from making so many beds and scouring all those sinks. I still marvel at the efficacy of my exercises.

One morning as I was washing windows, the group leader came by and saw me squeezing my Windex bottle. She was a good friend, and knowing that I was likely to be doing my work from my body's point of view, she started laughing. She said, "I know you're doing hand exercises, Darlene, but couldn't you wash the windows a little, too?" I suddenly realized that squeezing a nearly empty Windex bottle nearly 100 times before I got any Windex on the window was an unacceptable speed at which to get any window washing done. I was so focused on my exercises that I had lost sight of my work!

I don't advocate concentrating on the movements of your body to the detriment of your work, but I do want to suggest that one can become very good at doing both.

You can reverse a physical difficulty or heighten vibrant good health with a soul-satisfying combination of physical sensation and sense of accomplishment by living from the point of view of your body. You can practice this every day in your workday life. You can choose to take the body's point of view for a few hours a day, a few days a week, a few months at a time, a year, or as a more or less permanent point of view for the rest of your life. I encourage you to try it as an experiment. At the very least, you will increase your mental agility by going back and forth from goal-directed thinking and decision-making to registering feelings and sensations from different parts of your body. You may find that cerebral functions such as thinking and decision-making become clearer and easier once you pay attention to the body. That is because you will have a stable point of view from which to judge your possibilities. When people feel settled in their bodies, they frequently experience a clarity and certainty that is very helpful in arranging the priorities of their ordinary lives.

Chapter 6

Putting Together Your Treatment Plan

I f you find yourself debilitated in some way by the pain and stiffness of arthritis, it is wise to devise a treatment plan for yourself, to embark on it as soon as you can set up your life around it, and to continue for some designated period of time, perhaps six months. You can decide at the end of that period whether to continue with the plan the way it is or to change or eliminate some part of it, based on how you are feeling. You might decide, as I have, to continue most of the following plan for the rest of your life.

Diet

Although I noted earlier that I don't endorse rigid, restrictive diets, I think it is wise to monitor your daily food intake to the extent that you limit sweets, salt, fats, and meat—

foods that exacerbate swelling. In general, you should consume foods that are known to have antioxidant properties, such as vegetables in the broccoli family, supplementing these with legumes and easily digested grains. You should avoid overeating. At least eight glasses of clean water a day is a must. These practices ensure that the system is flushed and not deluged with material to be processed by an already overburdened body. If you are fairly conscientious about your diet most of the time, you can occasionally indulge yourself in some riotous sweet, a delectable starch sprinkled with salt, or a feast of meat.

For instance, in my own daily life I eat carefully. I try to include healthful foods in my diet every day, like grains, vegetables, and fruits. I'm conscientious about fluids and often carry water with me so that the swelling associated with my disease can be flushed. I try to avoid foods that seem to clog my system, like meat, sweets, salty chips, or too much of any food. Too much food leaves me feeling logy, as if my system were overburdened. I suspect that is exactly the case when I feel that way. My system, already encumbered with the task of carrying out normal bodily functions in the presence of inflammation and immune dysfunction, may well be overwhelmed with the prospect of digesting a huge meal. So I tend to eat lightly day to day. Rarely do I crave something I would prefer not to eat, like red meat or pastry. But when I do, I indulge that craving for a while, at least until it begins to seem a little habitual, like wanting a sweetroll for breakfast several mornings in a row. Then I will eat something else. If invited out to a restaurant, I usually order broiled fish or pasta, have a glass of wine, and top off the occasion with a truly wicked dessert. If I happen to go to a restaurant several nights in a row for some reason, I still order dessert but share it with others. If invited to someone's home, I eat whatever the host serves. Because I love all food and enjoy the fact that someone cooked it for me, there is nothing that I would refuse to eat in someone else's home. This is a truly special occasion for me, and I indulge myself totally in the pleasure of eating and the delight in being feted.

When it comes to diet, we're all different. What you need to do is observe your habits and cravings, the diet with which you function best, and then make a few (breakable) rules for yourself from those observations. It's actually more helpful to think in terms of *guidelines* rather than rules: For example, these are the circumstances under which I feel best; this is how often I need to violate those rules to enjoy myself; and so on. Some people dispense with having to observe and remember what they've been eating all the time by just instituting a system: They eat healthful foods during the week and splurge on the weekends. This seems like a good idea to me. I've been on that kind of weight-loss schedule, and it worked very well, leaving me with the feelings of having both taken care of my body and satisfied my love for rich food.

Exercise Session

This is an important daily ritual because it loosens the joints. I suggest scheduling this ritual whenever you tend to be stiffest, in the morning or in the evening. I am stiffest in the morning. I begin loosening my joints while I am still in bed with some basic stretches of my hips and shoulders. Then I do a series of exercises that help make grooming and dressing more comfortable for me and that prepare me physically—and mentally—for the day ahead. (For details, see chapter 7.) If you have osteoarthritis, your stiffest time may be at night, after a day of activity. In that case, an exercise session to ease the pain and stiffness accumulated during the day will feel the best. Some people are surprised when I prescribe exercises for the period of the day when they feel worst—they think that exercises are only for when you feel good—but that is because I am prescribing movements that loosen the joints and ease pain, not vigorous exercises that exacerbate it. When I talk about an exercise session, I am talking about working specifically on your pain and restriction, doing movements that reduce pain and increase mobility. I don't think anything is better for pain and stiffness than gentle movement; it's more effective than not moving at all. (If necessary, refer back to chapter 4, which gives guidelines on exercise movements and strategies.)

As for the amount of time to be spent doing movements, I recommend that you give your body some priority while continuing to maintain your daily life. I think three to five hours a day are necessary for extreme cases and dire situations. That is when you must focus your life on your body to the exclusion of other pursuits, or you will lose a great deal of mobility and control over your disease. After you have deterioration under control, an hour a day for maintenance is good.

Challenging Activity

Do some challenging activity a couple of times a week—anything that *challenges* your system, muscles, and joints, but without straining or harming them. You feel better afterward, stronger, more in control, the master of your fate. You know that you have chosen an activity that is too difficult for you if you feel too tired, achy, or discouraged. You should feel tired and tested but also stimulated and triumphant.

By doing a challenging activity a couple of times a week, you keep yourself on the frontier of your abilities with an eye to expanding them, rather than continually functioning well within your range of motion. Taking on and meeting a challenge successfully is a tremendous boost physiologically and psychologically. All your systems work better, your muscles, nerves, and brain are stimulated, and you have a higher opinion of yourself. It may take you a while to figure out what is challenging and what is too much for you, but it's worth the effort. *Hint:* Look at your activities from your body's point of view.

In chapter 9 we'll look at popular leisure activities, such as walking and biking, that can challenge your body—and serve as a source of pleasure.

Pleasure and Deep Relaxation

An ideal life is one in which nearly all of your days include activities that give you a sense of accomplishment interspersed with something that brings you pleasure. I put deep relaxation in the same category as pleasure because I believe the two have similar beneficial effects on the central nervous system. Moreover, as noted earlier, scientists have established a link between positive emotional states and enhanced functioning of the immune system. For most of us, the activities that bring us pleasure are those that take us into the realm of no time pressures, no responsibility—just ease and enjoyment.

Whatever you enjoy, try to do it as often as you can. Now that you are sick and your life has become a treatment plan for your recovery, you must prioritize your activities according to their beneficent effects on your body. If you are a stranger to pleasure and relaxation, consult people who can help you discover this part of yourself and its deeply healing effect.

Movement in the Water

Visit a pool a couple of times a week. It is important to find a pool (with warm water, if possible) in which you can perform motions that are too straining for you to do easily on land. You keep your body fluid and strong enough for your daily activities by periodically doing movements that you never do otherwise. Letting your legs float up alongside your hips or using your inner and outer thigh muscles to propel yourself across a pool makes your leg muscles stronger and stabilizes your joints, so that an activity like walking around the grocery store becomes easier and more pleasant. Nowhere else besides a pool can you recapture the feeling of lightness and ease that you experienced in your prearthritic body. This sensation is important to your well-being. (Swimming pool activities are covered in detail in chapter 9.)

Massage

Before you go to sleep, massage your body to work out the aches and pains that have accumulated during the day and to relax you totally for a deeply refreshing sleep during the night. If you discipline yourself enough at first to incorporate massage into your bedtime ritual, you'll soon find that it's one of the most pleasant things you do for yourself. (See chapter 7 for instructions.)

Have a professional massage every week if possible, or at least every other week. This may seem like too much self-indulgence to some people, but they overlook the physical benefits of receiving a massage. A professional massage increases allover circulation in the body, stimulates nerves and the regulatory systems of the body, and loosens the joints. Very few medical treatments do all that and feel so good at the same time. If your masseuse or masseur also moves your joints while you relax them during your session, your brain has the experience of your joints moving easily and effortlessly, an experience that can be generalized when you get up off the table. This is passive movement, which, as we have seen, is extremely powerful in its pain-relieving, nerve-stimulating effects. Your body has the experience of moving without pain or effort.

In choosing a masseuse or masseur,

choose someone you feel comfortable with and who treats your body with respect and care. If the person seems to be on automatic pilot, running off a standard technique on your body as if it were a piece of furniture, don't go back. You need special, individualized care, and you should insist on it. If you find someone who seems to relate to your body with sensitivity, feel free to instruct him or her during your sessions about what makes you feel good and what is painful. You should get up from a massage feeling relaxed and more mobile. It is also possible that you'll be sore the first few times because your body is not accustomed to being stimulated in this way. If the soreness persists past the first few times, however, your masseuse/masseur may be too rough. Either ask for more gentle treatment, or find a new masseuse/masseur.

*   *   *

The above suggestions for a self-healing treatment plan may be followed exclusively and gradually personalized as you become familiar with your own body, or they can be interspersed with your physician's recommendations and medical care. I believe they are conducive to a happy, healthy, normal lifestyle with minimal pain and restriction. Still, it is important to keep individual differences in mind. Some aspects of this plan may be more or less important for you. The main thing is to get in touch with your own body, your own rhythms, and your own needs and take whatever suggestions seem to apply to you and leave the rest. Now is the time for you to regard all aspects of your life as a giant buffet table from which you may choose what you personally want and need to find relief from pain and live in peace with arthritis.

Part II

EXERCISES FOR EVERYDAY LIFE

Chapter 7

Personal Care: Self-Reliance for Stiff Bodies

Before Getting Out of Bed . . .

When you wake up, while still in bed, lie on your back with your legs outstretched and check out each body part (e.g., toes, ankles, knees, hips, hands, upper back, shoulders, neck, and jaw) by moving it a little: jiggling it, wiggling it, turning it slowly. Open and close your hands slowly while moving your head from side to side. Then lift each shoulder, one by one, and let it sink back down onto your bed. Stretch your hips by pushing your legs out away from your body, one by one. Wiggle your toes.

How is your breath? Concentrate for a few minutes on what stiff people need more than anything else: breath going in and out of their bodies and subtly moving small muscles that gently expand the spaces between the joints. Breathe into your shoulders, breathe into your chest, your abdomen, your legs. Feel your chest gradually expand as you inhale and get smaller as you exhale. Feel your back expand as you inhale and get smaller as you exhale. Feel your legs lengthen as you breathe in and then out.

Put your hands on your stomach, and feel it rise and fall as you breathe. Soothe your stomach and your hands and encourage the breath. Feel the space between the bones get a little larger as you inhale. Feel your muscles gently settle around your joints as you exhale.

Now it's time to do some wave breathing. Continue the wave breathing until your body feels awake and supple.

Now slowly stretch in bed to accommodate the changes your breathing has brought. Feel that your legs are a little longer, your feet a little warmer. Don't be alarmed if you have a little involuntary shaking or trembling with this — it's just that your nerves are waking up and your blood is flowing back out to sleepy limbs.

After completing these preliminary movements, you are ready to perform the following exercises.

Exercises

ARM ROTATIONS OVER CHEST. While still on your back, stretch your arms out in front of your chest and interlace the fingers of your hands. Let your hands start leading your arms in rotating motion around your chest. Your arms can be very relaxed if you let your hands lead the motion. Feel your shoulders and neck relax as a result of your hands leading the motion; your hands take all responsibility for holding up your arms, for changing direction, for soothing your upper body. As you move, feel your shoulders and upper back gradually come back to life, as if they were being massaged by the movement. Change the direction of your rotation. Feel your breath expand your chest. Feel your shoulders fall back. Feel your neck flatten out against your pillow.

ADDITION OF HEAD MOVEMENT. Now that your arm motion is well established, begin to move your head slowly from side to side. Relax your neck; let your head move your neck. Move your neck easily, gently, from side to side, and feel it settling onto your pillow as your head moves slowly. Feel as if some wonderfully kind and benevolent person has taken your chin in her hands and is gently moving your head from side to side.

You are easily doing two different motions: rotating your arms around your chest, and moving your head from side to side. This is very good for your self-image if you think of yourself as a stiff person. Because different parts of your body are moving independently, your brain begins to think how loose you are. More and more you feel the ease in your chest, shoulders, and neck, and even your jaw. Continue to breathe as you move.

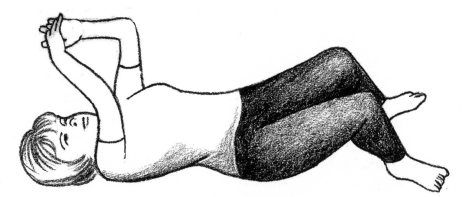

ADDITION OF ANKLE ROTATION. Now add one more movement: From the other end of your body, slowly rotate your feet around your ankles. Think of your big toe leading your foot around your ankle. Change the direction of your rotation from time to time. Now your brain is truly impressed! Doing all these intricate motions simultaneously, you are becoming looser and looser— possibly a lot looser than many of your more athletic friends are in the morning.

KNEE BENDS. Did your knees feel stiff or sore when you bent them for the first time this morning? Stretch them out on the bed again, and try bending them in a way that avoids early-morning stress on the knees: Take a deep breath and as you slowly exhale, imagine that your feet are bringing your knees upright. Imagine that as your feet move closer to your body, they are causing your knees to bend and come into an upright position. Let your feet work to move the knees. This emphasis on the feet working to put the knees in place rather than the knees

being dragged by the torso is very important in loosening the body and preparing it for the day.

HIP LIFTS. On your back, with bent knees, take a deep breath and slowly let it out. As you exhale, lift your right hip—only your right one—and feel it stretch out. Hold that stretch while you inhale. When you exhale again, drop that hip and lift the other one. Inhale again. Then, as you exhale, drop that hip and lift the other one. Do this easily, gently, with almost no effort. Lift with your breath, and let fall with your breath. Feel the stretch work itself up your back as you continue to move. Your thighs are working in this stretch. Let them work alone; relax your buttocks and upper body. Continue to stretch your hips alternately until your hips and lower back are looser and your thighs feel warm and strong.

SITTING UP. Now you're ready to sit up. Instead of using the "jackknife" method to jerk your body upright, turn over on your

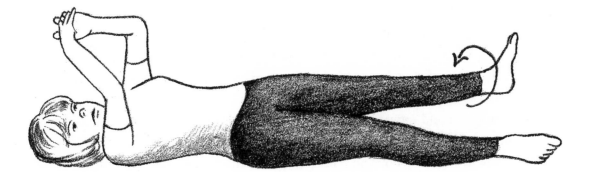

side and gently raise your body with your arms, while you breathe and your head and neck relax.

Sit on the edge of the bed in an easy, comfortable way, with your hands on your knees. Explore how your body actually *feels* to you, casting aside any preconceived notions of how it's supposed to feel. As you sit, feel all the parts of your upper body as they adjust to your upright posture: your head, your neck, your shoulders, your chest, and your midsection. Breathe deeply as you focus on each part.

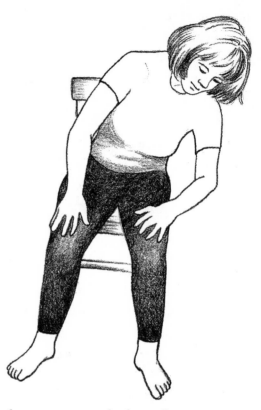

UPPER BODY ROTATIONS. As you feel your breath expand and fill your upper body, slowly rotate your upper body around your lower body, letting your neck fall forward when you go forward and letting your neck fall back when you go back. Move gently and slowly enough that the rhythm of your breathing is not disturbed. The rhythm of this motion should be the same as the rhythm of your breathing. As you continue to move, feel your upper body begin to separate more and more from your lower body; your legs are settled and still while your upper body becomes more and more mobile. Feel the muscles in your thighs relax and give way to the free motion of your upper torso. Lead this wide motion around your hips with your head rather than with your shoulder as you move backward and forward. Let your shoulders relax and separate from your neck and chest. Now change direction and repeat the movement, rhythmically rotating your upper body around your lower body. Finally, stop and sit with your hands on your knees and feel what you have accomplished with your movement. Feel the parts of your upper body again: your head, your neck, your shoulders, your chest, and your midsection.

FOOT STAMPING. While sitting on the edge of the bed, you can prepare your lower legs and feet to accept your weight before you actually get up by doing the following: Lift your feet, one at a time, off the floor, knees bent. Allow your hips to relax and your feet to do the work of lifting. Bring each foot back down again onto the floor in a quick, light way, one after the other, so that you are stamping the floor lightly with your feet. Keep the pressure of your feet on the floor well within comfort level.

ANKLE FLEXION AND EXTENSION. Sit on the floor or in a chair with your feet on the floor or on a comfortable cushion. Stretch your toes as far toward your shins as possible, imagining that your toes stretch so far that they elongate the whole foot toward your leg. Breathe deeply as you stretch.

While continuing to breathe deeply, stretch your foot out away from your shin

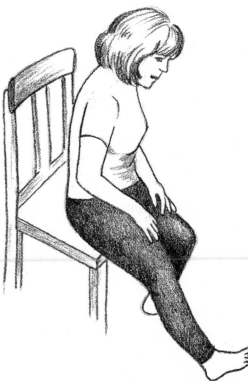

toward the floor as far as you can, imagining that your foot arches away from your leg and elongates toward the floor. Do this slowly and precisely. Continue to alternate flexing and extending. If one feels noticeably different from the other, try doing this exercise one foot at a time for a change.

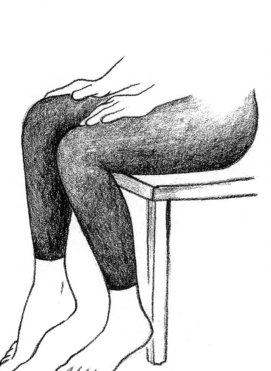

LIFTING AND STAMPING THE FEET. Once again, lift the feet. Your right foot lifts your right leg and comes down; your left foot lifts your left leg and comes down. Then do some light stamping of the feet to get blood down there and prepare the feet for standing. You should stamp the floor with the bottoms of your feet, one foot after the other, quickly, lightly, without any pain or stress on your feet or ankles. Now lift your knees together, push down against the floor, breathe out, and you're up!

Grooming

In the course of your daily functioning, you determine what activity you will perform, such as walking to the bathroom and taking a shower, but after the decision has been made, the movement itself will be executed best if you allow your body to tell you how to do it. If you switch into a *feeling* mode, you can feel the way your body tells you to move. How do you switch into this mode? Loose, pain-free movement has two major characteristics: (1) The rhythm of movement follows the rhythm of breathing—you perform a movement while your primary attention is on your breathing; (2) the parts of the body farthest from the torso lead the parts closest to the torso (i.e., feet lead legs, legs lead hips, hands lead arms, arms lead shoulders, head leads neck, and so forth), so that the feeling is one of expansion into the world, in contrast to the kind of contraction in which energy is drawn into the torso and held close so that the muscles of the hands, feet, legs, and arms are contracted into the torso with the resulting tightness and stiffness.

Showering

As you prepare for your shower in the morning, feel your hands pull off your night-clothes. Your foot leads you into the shower, under the warm, soothing water. Use the shower for a massage: Let the water beat hard on your chest as you breathe in and out for a few breaths; then let it beat on your thighs and the back of your neck. Take a deep breath, lower your chin onto your chest, and let the water beat onto your upper back as you breathe in and out. Use your back muscles to push your vertebrae out to meet the stream of water. Take a deep breath, put your chin on your chest again, and on the out-breath bend over enough to allow the spray to reach your lower back. Release the muscles being pummeled by the water.

Stretch out your arms away from your torso, and reach for the shampoo. Lather your hair, allowing your head to be moved on your neck, your elbows jutting out on either side. Feel your fingers on your scalp. Relax your neck as you move your head with your fingers. Let your shoulders fall away from your head. Feel their independence from your elbows. Caress/massage your body with the soap, your hand leading your arm.

As you bend your neck backward to rinse your hair, massage the back of your neck with your fingers. Gently move your chin forward and backward, about an inch or so in either direction. Your bobbing chin gradually extends the distance you can bend your head backward while you rinse.

Beat your hips and buttocks with loosely held fists to shake them alive as the water splashes over them. Place one hand on the inside and the other hand on the outside of your thigh, and shake it vigorously. Then shake the other thigh. Feel the shaking loosen the muscles of your thighs and buttocks.

Your hands reach for the sky as you rinse your underarms. Your chin rises as you rinse your face. Meet the water with your skin, breath, and bones. Feel its warmth and vitality penetrate all the way through to your tension and pain.

As you towel off, begin to notice where pain and tension persist, what movements cause discomfort. These are the places that need more attention. You must *feel* your aches and pains in order to ease them. It is useful to observe what kinds of movements increase or decrease your comfort and whether you can alter these movements enough during the course of your activity to affect your comfort level.

Brushing Teeth

Notice how you do the everyday, routine activity of brushing your teeth. Do you unconsciously grip the toothbrush in a stranglehold that precludes the loose, easy working of your fingers or wrist? Are your shoulders up around your ears? Do your shoulders and back do more work than your wrist and forearms? Do you hold your head forward while contracting your neck? Do you hang over the sink from your midback? If you have any of these constricting habits, you're working too hard to perform this simple task.

Here's what you should do to loosen up: Sit down and take a folded towel (pillow, mat, whatever) onto your lap so that you can put your elbows on it without bending forward. Your hands and wrists are loose, dangling from your forearms. Slowly rotate your hands around your elbows with your hands leading the motion. Breathe in and out naturally so that your breathing and the movement of your forearms are compatible. Breathe naturally; don't hurry your breathing to catch up with your arms. Do this motion until you are more aware of your hands and wrists than you were before. Feel your shoulders, neck, and chest relax as you breathe in and out.

Go back to the sink, pick up your toothbrush, and brush your teeth, your hand leading your forearm, while both shoulders are loose and fall away from the ears. Breathe deeply into your chest. Stand straight and tall. Now put down the toothbrush. Pick up your cup with your hand and forearm only (not your shoulder), fill it with water, bring it to your lips, and rinse your mouth. Feel the weight of your head as you bend forward to spit out the water. Push your vertebrae out one by one as you bend, first the vertebrae in the back of your neck, next between your shoulders, then between your shoulder blades, and finally in your midback. Feel the difference between each vertebra as you bend forward and come back up.

Feel your arm hang from your shoulder as the water splashes over your hand. Feel the roughness of the towel against your lips as you wipe your mouth. Experience a morning filled with sensations and textures. Brushing teeth can be a sybaritic delight.

Shaving

As you lather your shaving cream or lift your electric razor to your face, think about your body. Where is your breath? Does it expand the muscles of your chest or not? Are you using your shoulders and upper back as well as your hands to lead the razor around your face? Are your jaws held tensely? Does your neck ache?

The following is a simple exercise you can do to become increasingly aware of the distinctions between chest, shoulders, neck, and jaws while relaxing these body parts. After doing the exercise, you'll be able to shave more comfortably. Remember to stand as straight as you can, with relaxed shoulders and neck, and let your razor lead your hands around your face.

UPPER BODY DELINEATION. Rest your left hand on your knee or thigh. Put your right hand on your chest, fingers outspread, and begin to gently massage your chest, moving your hand in a small circle over the surface of your skin or nightshirt. Feel from the point of view of your chest what it feels like to be massaged. Feel from the point of view of your hand what it feels like to touch your chest. Breathe in and out, taking deep breaths. Feel your chest relax under your fingers.

Continue to massage your chest with your right hand. Very slowly, very gently, begin to rotate your left shoulder in small circles. (Your left hand is still resting on your knee or thigh.) Move your left shoulder in rotating motion while your other hand continues to massage your chest. Think of the *tip* of the shoulder as leading the motion, so that your neck can relax. The circles of rotation don't have to be very large; what is important is that your shoulder is gently moving while your chest is being soothed by your hand. Change the direction of your shoulder rotation. Feel the distinction between your chest, which is being passively massaged, and your shoulder, which is actively rotating.

While continuing to massage your chest and rotate your shoulder, begin to slowly move your head from side to side at the same time, leading the motion with your chin. This is a very gentle, very small movement: Your head moves slowly from side to side while your neck relaxes. Move the focus of your attention from chest to shoulder to neck and back again. Enjoy the loose feeling that results from these distinctions you are increasingly aware of between your upper body parts. Continue to breathe deeply. Notice the increasing independence of your neck, shoulder, chest, and arm.

Stop moving and sit quietly for a minute, your hands in your lap, feeling what your movement has accomplished. Notice the difference between the two sides of your upper body.

Now begin to massage your chest with your left hand while your right hand rests on your knee or thigh. Very slowly, very gently, begin to rotate your right shoulder in small circles. Move your right shoulder in rotating motion while your other hand continues to massage your chest. Change the direction of your shoulder rotation. Feel the distinction between your chest and your shoulder.

While continuing to massage your chest and rotate your shoulder, begin to slowly move your head from side to side at the same time, leading the motion with your chin. Your head moves from side to side slowly, while your neck relaxes. Move the focus of your attention from chest to shoulder to neck and back again. Enjoy the loose feeling that results from this movement, and notice the independence of your neck, shoulder, chest, and arm. Stop moving and sit quietly for a minute, your hands in your lap, feeling what your movement has done for your upper body.

Open and close your jaws a few times to relieve the tension there. Continue opening and closing your jaws until you feel more ease in the back of your neck.

Brushing and Combing Hair

Many people with arthritis have an especially hard time combing or brushing their hair. I cut my long hair when I first developed arthritis because it was so painful to lift my arms and make the long strokes required to get a brush through my thick mane. It was

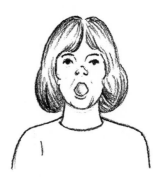

pretty difficult for me to watch my long waves fall to the floor of the hair salon, particularly because I was losing function in my shoulders and elbows. Is combing your hair as unpleasant an experience for you as it was for me then? Do you hurl an unwilling arm, buttressed by your rigid shoulder, into the air and then hold your breath until the excruciating process is over? Such a ritual of pain and contraction, not to mention the feelings of resentment and despair, can only further inflame painful joints.

It doesn't have to be this way. You can do what I have learned to do. Perform the following warm-up exercises and then use my step-by-step instructions to ease the process of brushing your hair.

ELBOW ROTATIONS AROUND SHOULDER. Sit down and put your hands in your lap. Breathe evenly and naturally. When you feel ready to move, bend your right elbow so that your hand comes up around your shoulder. Allowing your hand to dangle at the juncture of your shoulder and neck, raise your right elbow alongside your right ear. If this motion displaces your hand from your shoulder, don't worry about it. Allow your hand to dangle wherever it will when you raise your elbow alongside your ear.

Begin to rotate your elbow around your shoulder in large circles. Your elbow comes alongside your ear at one part of the rotation and points out away from your ear at another part of the rotation. Change the direction of your rotation from time to time. In this motion, the elbow leads, allowing the shoulder to relax while it is passively moved by the motion of the elbow.

Repeat with the left elbow.

SHOULDER ROTATIONS. Now rotate your right shoulder by itself. Think about the distance between your shoulder and your right ear. That distance gets less when your shoulder is at the top of the rotation. It gets greater when your shoulder is at the bottom of the rotation. Feel that distance change as you rotate. Change direction every once in a while so the rotation is forward as well as backward. Let your head adjust in whatever way it wants to while you rotate your shoulder. The muscles you are using to rotate your shoulder are also connected to your neck. You are affecting the tension level in your neck as well as in your shoulder as you move. Your neck wants to move in order to release that tension. Allow it to do so.

Repeat with the left shoulder.

ELBOW ROTATION. Finally, put a pillow on your lap at a height that allows you to place your elbows on your thighs without leaning over. If your vanity table is the proper height, you can use that surface. Your elbows are on either side of your body, resting on the pillow or table, with your lower arms up so that your hands hang loosely at the wrists. Begin to rotate your hands and forearms around your elbows, both arms at the same time. Your fingertips should lead the motion of your forearms around your elbow; allow your wrists to be loose. Your fingers are active and moving. Feel their effort as you move. Feel the tips of your fingers contact the cool air. Feel the bottom of your fingers where they join your palm. Feel your fingers lead the motion of your forearms around your elbows.

Continue to breathe and feel your shoulders, neck, and jaw relax as your arms continue to move.

STEP-BY-STEP INSTRUCTIONS. Focus your attention on your brush or comb, rather than your arms, as your brush or comb leads the strokes through your hair. Very slowly, as you exhale, let your brush or comb lead the motion of your arm. Let each out-breath support your arm in the air. Stroke only on the out-breath; rest your hand against your head on the in-breath if you need relief. Check to see that your shoulder is relaxed, that you are not tensing it unnecessarily. Let your shoulder fall on your out-breath in the same way you let it fall away from your ear while you were rotating it earlier. Inhale and feel your chest expand. Exhale and let your breath carry your stroke through your hair. Feel your neck, head, shoulders, arms, and wrists move separately as you breathe. Feeling your individual parts move is feeling loose.

Dressing

Pants/Slacks

People with stiff lower bodies develop complicated strategies for pulling on pants or slacks. Some stand, holding on to a chair for balance, and tug awkwardly at recalcitrant pant legs with one hand until they manage to heave them up to their waists and buckle them into place. This struggle is intended to avoid the conventional position, that of sitting on a chair and pulling up pants from the floor. If your legs seem too stiff to actively seek the opening at the end of the pant leg, or if your knees are too painful to bend, the conventional position seems too hard.

But the motions involved in the routine act of putting on one's pants are good exercises to activate the lower body and prepare it for walking and climbing stairs later in the day.

Notice when you sit on the edge of your chair, pants in hand, where in your body the restrictions are that give you difficulty with this task. Are your lower back and hips stiff?

Do you have weak legs or painful knees? The movements described here will help you deal with such problems.

THIGH SHAKE. Sit on the edge of your chair, and begin to vibrate/shake your upper thighs with your hands as you did in the shower. One hand rests on the inside of your thigh; the other rests on the outside of your thigh. With your hands in this position, give your thigh a good shake. Then shake the other thigh.

RAISE AND LOWER BENT LEGS. Still sitting, allow each foot to lift each leg alternately. Your knees remain bent. First your right foot lifts your right leg; then your left foot lifts your left leg. The motion is quick and light. Your feet are lifting your legs. You are not dragging them up by the hips. Let your hips relax against the chair. Lift your legs only as high as your feet can comfortably lift them, even if it is only an inch or two off the ground. It's more important to maintain the quick, light feeling than to go for range in this movement. Continue until you feel a little more life in your legs. Sit still for a few moments, and feel the sensations you have created in your legs and hips.

LEG ROTATION AROUND HIP, SITTING. Now with your hands on your right knee, guide your knee in a slow rotation around your hip. This means that as you rotate your

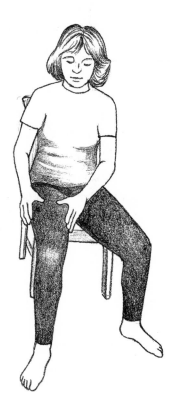

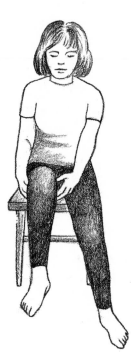

knee, your thigh is moved by the rotation of your knee only. Your foot remains stationary on the floor. Change the direction of the movement occasionally. Then repeat with the left knee, rotating first in one direction, then the other.

KNEE ROTATION IN CHAIR.   After your knees and hips feel a little looser, lift your right leg with your foot by putting your hands together behind the knee. Rotate your foot around your knee. This means that your foot rotates your lower leg in a circle while your knee and thigh are stationary. After a few

minutes let your foot come to rest again on the floor. Lift your left foot and hold it in the air as you rotate your foot around your knee. Continue until your left leg feels as stimulated as your right. Sit quietly for a breath or two, and feel the warmth in your legs.

To put on your pants: From a sitting position, take pants in hand, stretch your arms out toward your feet, and breathe deeply. As you breathe, let one foot find its way into one pant leg. Now the foot gently lifts your leg off the floor as you pull your pant leg over your leg. Now stretch out toward your other foot. Allow your out-breath to carry your

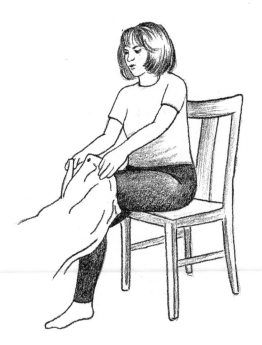

BREASTBONE FLEX. Sit quietly with your hands on your knees and breathe. When you inhale, allow the breath to rise from your diaphragm up into your chest and feel your chest muscles expand. When you exhale, feel your chest fall and sink as the air is expelled. Repeat this a few times until you are aware of your breastbone rising with each in-breath and falling with each out-breath. Now take a deep breath, hold it (don't exhale right away), and use your chest muscles to move your breastbone forward and back. Just your breastbone alone, without the participation of your shoulders or lower back. You can put your fingers on your breastbone to make sure that that is what is moving. When you need to exhale again, do so. Then, without inhaling right away, use your chest muscles to move your breastbone back and forth. This may be only a tiny movement, barely perceptible, if your chest is stiff and not used to moving without the help of other body parts. That's fine; it's better to move only your breastbone just a tiny bit than to move it farther with the help of other muscles. Isolating it will gradually make it loose and strong.

other foot into the pant leg. Take a new breath, breathe out gently, and pull on your pants. Stand and finish the task.

Sweaters

Pulling on a sweater is so ordinary, we don't realize how supple the upper body must be to do this gracefully. We all know the awkward feeling when we get "stuck" in a sweater midway on or off. You can't see; you can't reach; you feel helpless. Some of us routinely ask for help when pulling a sweater on or off. But as with pants or slacks, putting on a sweater is an excellent opportunity to perform the very motions that increase the feeling of mobility and breadth in our upper bodies.

If you cannot move your breastbone without using other parts of your body, continue your movement and, one by one, try to eliminate the parts of your body that are moving besides your breastbone, until at least you have that single, powerful, and perhaps very subtle movement of your breastbone alone, pushing out your chest and then collapsing toward your spine. Repeat the exercise several times.

ELBOW SWING. Cross your arms so that each hand rests on the opposite elbow. Your thumbs are resting on the inside of the opposite elbow, and your fingers are resting on the outside of the opposite elbow. If your fingers do not reach all the way to your elbows, rest them on your forearms. Now with your elbows leading, begin to swing your arms gently from side to side, your hands still resting comfortably on your elbows (or forearms). Breathe naturally during this motion,

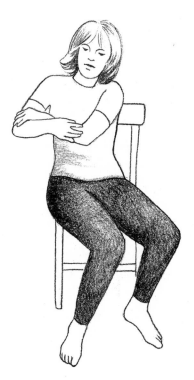

and your breath will help the motion loosen your shoulders and upper back. If you are loose enough, your motion will begin to twist your torso gently as you swing your elbows. Let that happen. Your head will also want to follow your elbows. This is fine. For a little extra twist in the neck, turn your head in the opposite direction from your arms. Continue until you feel some ease in your upper back. When you are finished swinging, put your hand on your knees and breathe. Feel the sensations you have created in your back and neck.

ARM ROTATIONS AROUND CHEST. Sit comfortably with your hands on your knees and breathe. Interlace the fingers of your two hands together in front of your chest, and raise your interlaced hands in the air, allowing your arms to be loose and comfortable. Begin to rotate your arms around your upper body. It is important that your hands lead the motion and that your arms and shoulders are loose and relaxed. Your shoulders relax as your hands lead your arms in rotation around your chest and head. The range of your rotation should be small at first until you feel your shoulders loosen up; then you can extend your range of motion.

Change direction occasionally, being careful to let your hands lead the change, not your arms or shoulders. Check that your shoulders, neck, and jaw are completely relaxed and are not involved in the rotation of your hands and arms around your upper body.

CHEST CIRCLES. With your upper body looser and more alive, you may feel the heaviness and tension in your arms. Put your hands on your chest. Take a deep breath, and on the out-breath, extend both arms in front of you, palms down, and move your arms apart in a circular motion away from each other toward your sides. Let your hands lead the motion.

Your hands move back to the chest in a circular motion that will bend your arms. Then, as your hands go out in front of you again, your arms are extended. Each arm moves in a circle on either side of your body. This is how the arms move during the breast-stroke in swimming. Again and again your hands extend your arms out in front of you, leading your arms in a circle, then back to your chest. Because your hands are leading, your shoulders are relaxed. You have a sense of your hands holding up your arms easily as they move. Inhale and feel your chest expand as your arms move out away from your body. Exhale as your hands return to your chest before your arms spread out again. It feels as if your hands have all the responsibility for the movement of your arms. Let your shoulders and upper back relax. After you have done this motion several times, return your hands to your knees. Sit quietly, and feel the vitality in your upper body.

To pull on your sweater: Pick up the garment, insert your hands in either sleeve, and make the broad sweep with your arms that you just finished doing. Pull the sweater over your head. Push your chest forward, extend your elbows, and grasp the bottom of the sweater to pull it down. Adjust its fit by pushing your breastbone back and forth until it feels comfortable. You might notice how energized your upper body feels.

Buttons, Snaps, and Hooks
To button, snap, or hook your clothing, your hands must be agile, and you must be able to feel subtle differences in the objects that you touch. If your fingers feel stiff and clumsy, you can make them more mobile by exercising them. Begin with a massage. Use the fingers of your right hand to massage your left fingers. Massage each finger briefly, taking mental note of any pain or restriction that you feel in the knuckle or joint. Next, gently rotate each finger around its knuckle, taking care to stay well within its range of motion so as not to cause pain. This aware-ness of each finger's range of motion will greatly develop your sense of its potential over the long run. Last, stretch each finger backward just to the point of pain but not beyond; then bend it forward toward the

palm of the hand. Switch hands and work on the right fingers in the same way. Over time you will come to know each one of your fingers as an individual with its own restrictions, pleasures, and potential. You don't have to consciously think about how each one functions as you use your hands, but the information you derive from moving each finger during your exercise time will be used by your nervous system as you go about your daily tasks. Your brain continuously processes hundreds of thousands of bits of kinesthetic information from your body, much more than you could consciously direct. Working on your hands greatly increases the stimulation your brain receives from them.

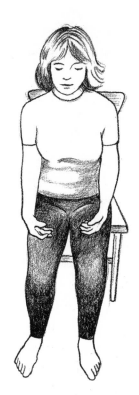

Now that your hands are less stiff, place them palms up on your knees or let them lie loose and relaxed at your sides as you sit. Very slowly bend your fingers in toward the palm of your hands so that your fingertips touch the skin. Then very slowly open your hand so that your fingertips stretch out into the air. Open and close your hands in this way several times. Feel the contact of each fingertip on the palm of your hand as you close your hands. Feel the cool air on your fingertips as you open your hands. See if you can open and close your hands so slowly that your fingertips become sensitive enough to "sense" the palm of your hand *before* they actually touch it. When your sense of touch has become this subtle, move your fingers immediately to your buttons and see if your sensitivity makes the task of buttoning any easier. Feel the smooth edge of each button. Feel the comparatively rough texture of the buttonhole of your shirt. Feel the raised surface of the threads around the buttonhole. Pass the button through the hole, and be totally aware of all the edges that facilitate the fit.

Shoes and Socks/ Stockings

However you put your shoes on—by bringing your feet up to your hands as you sit in a chair or by stretching your hands over your knees to reach your feet—you need to bend your spine to bring your hands and feet together. This is unfortunate if you feel your spine as a rigid, unyielding part of your body. But dressing your feet can be a daily exercise if you wish to make your back more pliant. You can put on your shoes and socks by sitting in a chair and bending your knees so as to bring your feet within range of your hands. Or you can stand and put each foot in turn on the seat of a chair so that you can reach your feet by bending over your knees.

SPINE CURL IN CHAIR. Sit in a chair with your hands on your knees. Breathe deeply into your belly a few times, and become aware of your back. What part of it is holding you up? Notice whether your back is moved at all by your breathing, and if so, what part of it you can feel when you breathe. Take a deep breath, and on the out-breath put your chin toward your chest, all the way onto your chest if you can. Then take another deep breath, and on the out-breath begin to bend over toward your knees. Bend vertebra by vertebra. Make this movement as much like curling up as you possibly can, so that all the vertebrae in your upper back are stretched, not just one or two. Come back up and try it again, stretching your elbows out from your sides and curling up as you drop toward your knees. Breathe in this position, and feel the different vertebrae of your back. If there is pain anywhere in your back, try to push out against the vertebrae just above and just below the pain so that the painful place will have the support of neighboring vertebrae.

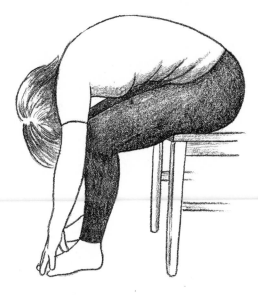

Bend several times until you are more aware of your spine and back muscles.

SIDE SPINE CURL OVER KNEES. Now take another deep breath, and on the out-breath drop your chin onto your chest and bend over your left knee, letting your arms drop down to your feet if they will reach that far. Come up on the next out-breath. Take another deep breath, and on the out-breath drop your chin onto your chest and bend over your right knee, letting your arms dangle and touch your feet if they will reach that far. Come back up. Now try bending over your knee in the same way to pull on your sock and shoe.

SPINE CURL OVER KNEE WITH CHAIR. If you choose to put each foot in turn on the seat of a chair, do the bending exercise in the same way from a standing position. Take a deep breath. On the out-breath, allow your chin to drop onto your chest. Then bring your hands together over your head. Stretch out your arms toward your feet as you bend over your knee. Breathe deeply, and continue to stretch your vertebrae on the out-breath. You can treat putting on your socks and shoes as a part of the exercise. Continue to breathe and stretch as you adjust your shoe. Repeat with the other foot. Now stand in your shoes, and feel the sensation in your spine, down your legs, and into your feet nestled in your shoes.

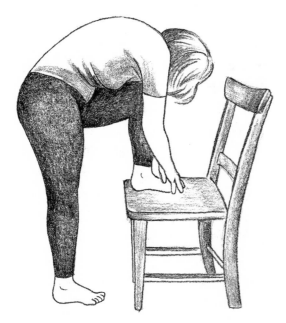

Surrendering to the Pillow and Bed

If you have any kind of degenerative condition, it becomes extremely important to get a good night's rest. It can be very difficult to get enough rest if you are having a painful flare-up or if your joints customarily ache during the night.

If you have difficulty sleeping because of discomfort caused by arthritis during the night, it may be helpful to you to approach bedtime with some ease-inducing rituals.

Self-massage

Even if you have never given a massage in your life, you can do a great deal to ease your pain and the day's physical and mental stress by massaging yourself in bed before you settle down for the night. You may wish to take a warm bath and/or drink a hot beverage before you start the massage. Or you can put your glass on the nightstand and take sips of your drink while you massage your neck, your hands, your arms, your knees, and especially your feet.

Self-massage should be done gently so that the area being massaged and your hands and arms feel relaxed and soothed by the effort. If you exert yourself so much that you are exhausted after massaging a part of your body, it seems like wasted effort.

To massage your neck, incline your head slightly to the right side and tap gently on the left side of your neck and shoulder with the fingertips of the right hand. Your hand reaches across your body and taps your neck

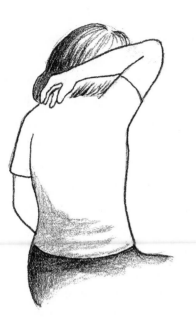

them, feeling for swollen areas and gently pinching these areas to encourage the excess fluid back into the bloodstream. You can also gently massage the muscles of your forearms and upper arms with the cream. Again, gentle touch will best prepare you for a night's sleep. You don't want to exert yourself or rough up the areas you are massaging. Ease and pleasure are your goals.

Spending five minutes apiece on each knee and each foot will repay you again and again in the increased ease of these parts during the night and even when you put weight on them again the next morning. Plus your hips will feel better if your knees and feet are relaxed instead of cramped and aching when you settle into bed. Knees and feet are best massaged with some lubricant like cream or oil. Again, it is up to you whether the oil is warm or cold.

Put a small amount of cream or oil on your knee, and gently begin to rub it in a circular motion. Your touch is more exploratory than insistent, for you are interested in feeling and soothing the bones and tissues of your knee. As with swollen elbows, you can reduce the swelling in your knee by gently pinching the swollen areas and encouraging the fluid to enter the bloodstream, thereby washing the fluid away. Along the inside of your knee you may be able to feel the stringy fiber of your ligaments. You can encourage them to receive blood by massaging them very gently. In all my experience with my own knees and the arthritic knees of clients, I have never found any-

and shoulder. When these muscles feel relaxed, incline your head to the left side and tap those muscles with the left hand. If you can reach the nape of your neck, you can tap or rub it soothingly with the fingertips of both hands.

If your hands ache, you may want to massage them in a bowl of warm water. If they are very swollen, cold water may feel better than warm. You may prefer to use cream or oil; I recommend that you use heating oil (oil containing wintergreen like Tiger Balm or Mineral Ice) or keep your oil in the refrigerator so that it is cold. You can make your hand massage brief, yet effective, by gently stroking each finger with comfort and pleasure in mind. If your elbows ache, you can also rub

thing more effective than massage for restoring pain-free movement to knee joints. If you put your knees to bed with a gentle massage that reduces swelling and eases pain, you will be more comfortable all night.

After working on both knees, proceed to your feet and ankles. They've supported you all day; now you can do a little something for them. I find the relief of my feet tremendously effective in easing my sleep. Put a little oil or cream on the top of your foot, and gently soothe your foot and ankle with one hand on the top of your foot and the other under the arch. One hand moves up toward the ankle, and the other explores the ball of the foot, under the toes. All feet love to be rubbed and soothed after a day's exertion. Intersperse massage with the gentle tapping of your fingertips on particularly tense or painful areas. This spontaneously releases the tension in the tiny muscles and is extremely soothing.

Sweet Dreams

When you are ready to put yourself to bed and to sleep, *feel* your body stretch out on the bed; *feel* your neck yield your head to the pillow. Be as aware as you can of the gradual letting-go process of the muscles of your body as they relinquish control. Breathe deeply and feel your chest and abdomen expand as air goes in, and feel the areas shrink as your breath goes out. Gently stretch your arms and legs, your hands and feet, away from your torso.

Breathe in and out and feel your head surrender to your pillow, your back surrender to your bed, your hips and thighs give up their control to relaxation. Feel each vertebra, each muscle in your neck and back give itself up to the comfort of your pillow and bed. If your eyes feel restless and unable to close, gently tap yourself on your forehead and around your eye sockets with your fingertips.

If you feel restless and tense in general, begin to expand each area of your body with your incoming breath, starting with the top of your skull and working down to your feet. Every time you inhale, imagine that your in-breath expands the part of your body you are thinking of, and when you exhale, imagine that that part of your body shrinks back to normal size. For instance, when you inhale, imagine that the top of your skull expands out to the walls of your room, and when you exhale, imagine that it returns to normal size. Next, imagine that your in-breath expands your forehead out to meet the walls of your room and that your in-breath returns it to normal size. Continue with your cheekbones, neck, shoulders, ribs, spine, hips, and so on, until you have expanded all your body parts down to your toes. You can return and concentrate on any parts that are particularly tense or painful. This is also a useful exercise if you should wake up in the middle of the night feeling anxious or uncomfortable.

If you find it difficult to concentrate enough to relax with all this breathing and imagery at first, don't be discouraged. It takes time to replace old habits with new, especially in the realm of thought. Be patient with yourself; give yourself plenty of time—at least a month or two—to test the effectiveness of these bedtime exercises. It's not easy to substitute new modes of thought for ones you've had for years, as you know if you've ever tried to stop biting your nails or give up smoking. Congratulate yourself on small successes at first, such as being able to relax your back a little more or finding it a little easier to rest your head on the pillow. Continue to massage and soothe your joints for the pleasure this provides. Practice your relaxation and visualization, and magnanimously let your body choose its own pace for settling down at night.

Chapter 8

Doing Household Chores Without Pain

In the Kitchen

Many people perform kitchen work at breakneck speed to get out of the kitchen as soon as possible. That's understandable when joints are sore and preparing a meal is painful and frustrating. Statistics show that nearly 40 percent of people with rheumatoid arthritis are malnourished because they find meal preparation such an ordeal. This is even more disheartening when you realize that kitchen work can be part of a healing strategy, as well as enormously satisfying, if you make the effort to break old habits and begin to perform your tasks from your body's point of view.

We spend so much time in the kitchen, even preparing very simple meals and cleaning up afterward, that it makes sense to turn kitchen work into a healing and productive activity.

Because many kitchen tasks require repetitive movements rather than heavy thinking, you can focus on turning food preparation and cleanup into a deeply satisfying relaxation-through-movement session. You can view all your activity from the point of view of your body and break down most of your tasks into tiny units of healing movement, each one of which you perform gracefully and precisely. In my kitchen, I feel that I'm as close to being a dancer as I'll ever be.

Reaching

Reaching for something on a shelf is an opportunity to stretch the arm out from the shoulders and body as if you were a dancer taking a position. Begin by breathing deeply and slowly. Focus on your fingertips as they reach toward the object you seek. Feel as if your fingertips themselves were pulling your arm right out of your shoulder and then your shoulder right out of your upper body. Allow your neck to fall back; your neck muscles are not needed to reach the object. Encourage your relaxed neck to separate itself from the effort your shoulder makes as your fingertips extend even farther. Feel the muscles along your side stretch. If you can rise on the balls of your feet, feel your calf and foot muscles contract to support your weight. If you're right-handed, don't always reach with your right side; give your left side a chance to experience this stretch as well.

The following exercise will help you prepare tight muscles along your side for a gentle stretch when you do it for the first time. Later on it will help you maximize the stretch after your ribs have become looser.

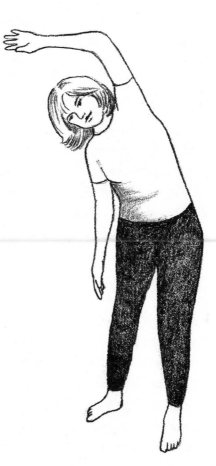

RIB STRETCH.   Stand with your feet slightly apart for a stable base. Let your arms hang loosely at your sides. Your knees are loose, not locked. Feel the crown of your head incline toward the sky. Raise your right arm, palm inside, straight over your head close to your ear. Begin to stretch that arm to the opposite, left, side of your body, over your head, and let your whole upper body gradually follow. Let your head fall to the left side as your body stretches. Let your body follow the lead of your arm gradually, stretching out under your right arm and pushing out your right side in an exaggerated way. Breathe deeply and regularly as you stretch, moving on the out-breath only, and your breath will protect you from stretching too far. It is important that all the muscles of your side be activated and share the burden of your stretch, not just the muscles around your waist. Now let your right arm bring you back to upright posture. Let your body follow the lead of your right arm. Repeat with your left arm and side.

Lifting

Since lifting heavy pots off the stove or carrying kettles full of water from the sink is so difficult and painful for arthritics, we usually set up our kitchens so as to minimize this activity. Dragging pots along a counter from the sink to the stove is helpful, as is carrying a large pot on the forearms rather than from the wrists. A certain amount of lifting in a kitchen is inevitable, however. The milk carton has to get from the refrigerator to the table; the cooked pasta has to be drained; the chicken has to be lifted from the oven. These chores can be demoralizing, but there are movements you can do before lifting heavy objects that can prepare your joints to take on a load with minimal pain (see below). Afterward, the same movements can relieve that wrenching you feel from unusual exertion.

I recommend the following procedure when you lift a heavy object: First take a deep breath, and as you exhale, lift the object. Then breathe up into your chest and straighten your spine as you carry it. Encourage your arms and upper back to carry the object rather than your shoulders and neck. Breathe deeply the whole time.

After you set the object down, let your arms fall to your sides and repeat the warm-up movements. If you feel aches or pains in your lower back, gently rotate your hips to stretch the little muscles around your spine.

ARM SHAKE. Stand with your feet slightly apart, for a stable base. Let your arms hang loosely at your sides. Starting from the tips of your fingers, begin to shake your arms in a loose, easy way. This should be gentle shaking, almost trembling, so it feels good rather than too vigorous for sensitive joints. Feel your arms shake out of your shoulder joints so that it feels like more space is created in those joints.

HAND SWING. Stand with your feet slightly apart, for a stable base. Let your arms hang loosely at your sides. When your arms are relaxed, interlace the fingers of your two hands together in front of you, at about thigh level. Begin to swing your two arms together, first to the right and then to the left, with your hands leading the motion. Your hands gently swing your straight arms from right to left, then from left to right. Let your torso swing, led by your arms. Even your head will want to follow your hands. Swing until your shoulders and arms feel warm and alive.

TOUCH SHOULDERS WITH FINGERS. Sit on the edge of a chair so that your feet rest securely on the floor. Extend straight arms out to either side away from your body. Bend both arms at the elbows so that the fingers of both hands touch your shoulders at the same time. Extend your arms again and repeat. Even if you can't reach your shoulders with your fingertips, you can loosen your wrist, elbow, and shoulder joints with this exercise.

Chopping, Mixing, Spreading, Washing Dishes

Everyone with arthritis is familiar with the difficulties encountered when one needs to perform tasks that require strength in the hands and forearms. If your fingers and wrists hurt or are inflexible, you begin to form the constricting habit of using parts of your body closer to your torso; that is, you use your upper arms, shoulders, and upper back as substitutes for forearms, wrists, and hands. Unfortunately, you soon feel the unpleasant results when chopping vegetables, mixing ingredients, or washing dishes: Your shoulders and neck ache or feel tense, perhaps even are acutely painful. Your upper spine feels contracted. No wonder you despair when it comes time to prepare meals.

The solution is to use the parts of your body that were meant to perform these jobs and let your shoulders, neck, and back relax. This may seem impossible to you if your fingers are very stiff, but you eventually may

be able to double their flexibility, and that would make your food preparation half as difficult. Plus, over time, your hands and forearms would become stronger.

I have found that a heavy knife is best for chopping and cutting in the kitchen, because its weight often is an effective substitute for the pressure of my wrist. When I pick up the knife, my hand feels the coldness of the stainless steel blade and the sculpted edge of the knife handle. My hand also feels the temperature and textures of all the food I pick up and touch. While I chop, I raise my forearm up and down in rapid strokes while the knife cuts efficiently through the food. Even with carrots or beets, I find I can chop easily and quickly with a minimum cost to my wrist and hands if my arm hangs loosely out of the shoulder joint.

When I clean up after meals, I apply the same principles. If I wipe off the table and wash the dishes with the emphasis on the movement of my hands and forearms rather than my neck and shoulders, I feel much better during and after my work. When I wash dishes, I try to be patient with myself, to take the time to move the washcloth gently over the dishes, to extend my fingers and wrists as needed.

You may want to begin your own kitchen work with a full massage of both hands as described on pages 155–57. This would make a pleasant beginning for work that is both necessary and possibly therapeutic. But if you feel impatient, perhaps you would rather just stretch out the individual fingers of each hand. Do each finger of one hand before going to the other hand. Use your left hand to stretch each finger of your right hand. Gently stretch the thumb and each finger one at a time, away from the palm of the hand, and then release them back toward the base of each finger. Don't take any joint beyond its ability to stretch. Go to the border of discomfort and come back. Then use your right hand to stretch each finger of your left hand in the same way. This stretching will warm your hands and prepare them for work.

The following exercises will isolate and stretch in turn your elbows, chest, shoulders, neck, arms—your whole upper torso—so that chopping, mixing, spreading foods, and washing dishes can be done more comfortably. Perhaps, as happened with more than one of my clients who did these exercises, such tasks will become possible for the first time in years. All these small, gentle movements to loosen up the joints in the chest, shoulders, arms, and neck can be done sitting down. Since standing at the kitchen counter or sink can be painful for the lower body as well, I've also included two exercises that work first the hips and knees and then the toes and heels.

ELBOW FLAP. Sit straight in a chair with your feet firmly on the floor in front of you.

Put your shoulders back, bend your arms, and attempt to touch your elbows together behind your back. It doesn't matter if your elbows don't actually touch; just the effort of bringing them together will stretch the muscles in the front of your shoulders and chest. To stretch the muscles in your upper back, bring your arms forward, with your forearms hanging down, and stretch your elbows toward each other, twisting your arms so that the *backs of your hands meet,* and your forearms twist toward each other. You know you are doing this correctly when you feel the stretch in your upper back. Touching your

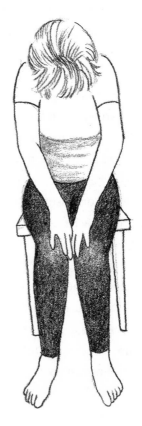

elbows together with your forearms up in front of your face may be easier (thus assuring your success), but attempting to touch your elbows together with your forearms down will supply a deep stretch you can feel in your upper back. Now bring your elbows together behind your back again. Then again in front. Do the motion with lightness and speed. Breathe normally, allowing your breath to go in and go out as you move. Continue to touch your elbows together in back and in front until you feel stretched in your upper back and chest. When you have become accustomed to moving your elbows forward and back, begin to let your head fall gently forward when you touch your elbows in front and let your head fall gently back when you touch your elbows together in back.

NECK STRETCH. Sit with your feet firmly on the floor. Put your hands together behind your head. Relax your neck and head, and with your hands, bring your chin to your chest. Raise your head up again. Bring your chin to your chest with your hands. Continue bringing your chin to your chest with your hands and raising your head up again until your head goes forward and backward on your neck more easily.

ARM TWIST. Let your arms dangle loosely at your sides. Turn your palms in toward your body and then out away from your body, twisting your arms in the process. You don't have to move your arms, just your hands and wrists. Your arms will follow the twisting motion of your wrists. Let your arms hang loosely at your sides while your hands do the work. This is a very gentle but stimulating exercise for sore elbows and tired arms.

ARM STRETCH ACROSS TABLE. Do one final stretch before you begin work. While sitting at your worktable, stretch your straight arms out from your shoulders across the table, allowing your head and upper body to rest on the table as well. Continue to stretch your arms out across the table, feeling the pull in your upper back and shoulders as you stretch. This is an excellent stretch to do midtask as well if you feel an accumulation of tension in your upper body.

HIP AND KNEE ROTATIONS. Stand with feet apart and begin to rotate hips, first in one direction, then in the other. Breathe normally, and allow the hips to move easily, separating from your upper body. There is no shoulder or upper body movement in this exercise. Your upper body relaxes while your hips move in rotation around it. After a minute or so, stop rotating the hips, and begin to rotate the knees, first in one direction, then in the other. Breathe normally, and allow your lower legs to lead a rotation around your knees. Your hips will move, too, but when you are rotating your knees, the hips are not the leader of the motion. Notice as you rotate your knees how your weight is distributed over your feet. Stop rotating your lower legs, and return to the hip rotation, noting how different it feels in your knees and in your feet. Return to the knee rotation, and again notice the difference between this and the hip rotation in terms of your knees and feet. This exercise is wonderful to do for ten minutes or so, and your lower back and leg joints will feel very different than if you had merely planted your legs on the floor as if they were sticks in the ground while you washed the dishes.

TOE/HEEL ROCK. Stand with feet apart. Rock forward onto your toes as far as you can. Breathe normally and relax your upper body as much as you can. Now rock backward onto your heels with your toes pointing up. Continue to rock forward and backward. This exercise relieves tension in your feet and strengthens the calf and shin muscles in your legs.

Housework

The ordinary demands of housework are a challenging workout for your body. As such, housework can either add to the strain and deterioration of an unhealthy body or be part of the program that makes you fit and energetic. It all depends on the way you choose to move while you exert your arms, legs, and back in your work. The old habit patterns tell us to rush through unpleasant tasks even if we must spend the rest of the day recovering. There is an alternative approach: You can choose to do housework from your body's point of view, giving priority to how your body feels while you work, no matter how long it takes. You might be surprised to find that over the long term, this is not so inefficient an approach as you originally thought. The recovery time afterward will be very short, and you will be pleased with how your body begins to feel while you are doing demanding work.

Dusting, Wiping, Polishing

While dusting shelves and furniture, wiping surfaces, and polishing tabletops, you can keep your shoulders, neck, and upper back limber if you move your arms in such a way that your upper body joints are loosened by your work. These cleaning activities require a lot of shoulder and upper back movement. It is most helpful if your hands lead all these motions of the arms; your shoulders are loosened by the movements of the hands and arms. Most of us use our right side exclusively for housework. Your left side needs movement, too, so while your right arm is busy dusting or wiping, try rotating your left arm in various directions so that when you are finished, you don't feel a great discrepancy between the right and left sides. Try using your left hand occasionally to dust or polish.

Begin your housework with a few loosening exercises. Then do your tasks from your body's point of view.

ARM CIRCLES. While standing or sitting, rotate your straight arms out in front of your body, making large circles, your hands leading the motion. The circles should be wide enough that your arms are drawn out to the sides of your body as well as in front. Rotate your arms in both directions in front of your body.

Next rotate your arms in wide circles from the sides of your body, each arm straight out from each side. It is important that your shoulders are relaxed and supported by your midback, that they are not up around your ears attempting to hold up your arms. If they feel as if they are supporting the weight of your arms, relax them by letting them fall with each out-breath.

If you cannot relax your shoulders while rotating your arms straight out from your body, rotate your straight arms at your sides with your hands at hip level, your shoulders and arms completely relaxed, your hands leading the motion. Rotate your arms in both directions.

ARM ROTATIONS BEHIND BACK. Because dusting, wiping, and polishing require your hands and arms to be in front of you for long periods of time, you need to relieve the strain on your neck and shoulders intermittently and use other muscles in your upper body. Pause periodically in your work to push your shoulders down and back, but don't tighten your arms. Allow your arms to continue to hang loosely from your shoulders. This relieves your upper back and shoulders from the strain of supporting your arms while they work. Rotate your straight arms in small circles behind your back, allowing your hands to lead the motion. Change the direction of your rotation from time to time. This feels good, and it is very good for your body to use a variety of muscles as you work rather than repeatedly straining the same ones.

CROSS ARMS IN BACK. Another exercise that relieves this kind of strain is to put your straight arms behind your back, palms up, so that the backs of your hands rest on your buttocks. Then begin to swing your arms behind you, first out from your sides and then back across each other in scissor fashion so that your hands cross in back. Breathe deeply so that your chest expands as your arms work behind you. This exercise is very relaxing.

ELBOW TWIST. Bend your arms out from your sides with your elbows out, your forearms hanging down, and your hands dan-

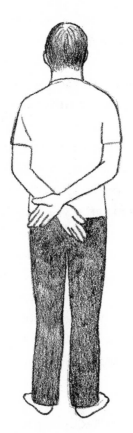

ments. Let your duster or cloth trace a rotating motion on the surface you are cleaning, so that your arms and shoulders are rotated in their joints by your cleaning motions. You can minimize the painful pressure of cleaning work on your wrists by distributing that pressure more evenly across your hand and fingers. Place the duster or cloth in your hand so that all the joints of your fingers take part in holding and using it. Even if such activity is extremely clumsy at first because you are not accustomed to using joints that have been stiff for some time, it is worthwhile to cultivate the patience necessary to begin using these joints again.

As you make gentle demands on these joints and the muscles around them, the nerves in them will activate and tell your brain that the joints and muscles need blood and nourishment again. This in turn will reduce your swelling and pain and make the joint more flexible. Your brain will respond more and more as you use the joint more and more. Your whole body and brain is a feedback system. If you use your hands and wrists, they will be nourished and their waste products (the swelling) will be taken away by the bloodstream. If they are not used, your brain will forget about them until you accidentally jerk them, causing pain.

gling loosely from your wrists. Let your elbows lead your upper body in a gentle twisting motion that relieves strain to your upper back. Don't hold your body against the movement; allow your body to follow your elbows as they swing around from side to side. When you are comfortable with this movement, you might allow your head to fall forward on your neck so that it, too, is being moved as you turn.

WORKING FROM YOUR BODY'S POINT OF VIEW. As you work, be conscious of your body, feeling the effect of all your movements.

When you are aware of your body as you work, you notice any tension that builds up in your neck and shoulders. To relieve the tension, repeat the arm movements suggested above. While you are tending to your body, your cleaning activity can continue at the edges of your consciousness. If you work from the point of view of your body, you can have a good workout for your shoulders, arms, and upper back and dust your furniture at the same time!

On the other hand, if you feel too stiff and achy to do the exercises suggested above, but you still feel compelled to get some housework done, you will benefit more from a very gentle arm movement (see below). If this movement makes your arms feel better, you can get up and begin to work, remembering to work from the point of view of your body, with your hands leading your arm motions. You can continue to exercise as you work, rotating your shoulders directly and tapping on your shoulders and neck muscles with your fingertips. If you work from the point of view of your body, your focus will be on how you feel with each movement rather than on how much work you are getting done, and you will be much less likely to add to your soreness. If you can concentrate on easing your discomfort by the way you move so that you actually feel better after you finish some housework, how delighted you will be. You will feel that you actually have some control over your life, that whatever obstacles your arthritis poses, you can cope with them and even remove them. If you move and work from your body's point of view, you'll be doing wonders for your situation.

The satisfaction that derives from reversing loss of function from a chronic illness is indescribable.

STRAIGHT ARM ROTATIONS AROUND SHOULDER. Lie on your side with both legs slightly bent, the top knee bent forward to the floor, if possible, for more stability. If you cannot reach the floor by bending your upper leg forward, it is fine to just rest your upper leg comfortably on your lower leg. Your head should be supported, either by your outstretched lower arm or by a pillow. Raise your upper arm straight into the air. Begin to rotate it in small circles around your shoulder, your hand leading the motion. Your hand leads the motion so that your shoulder and neck can relax. Your shoulder is passively moved by the motion of your arm; it is not making the motion happen. Feel the trapezius muscle in your neck and shoulder relax as you move your arm. Keep your rotational circles well within your range of motion so that you are not fighting gravity to do this movement. If your hand leads the motion, it will not tire you to rotate long enough to loosen and soothe your aching shoulder. It is important to stay on the frontier of your pain without actually going into it. Stay relaxed and comfortable, but rotate your arm in the area where movement is most restricted. Change the direction of your arm rotation from time to time. After you feel looser and less achy in your shoulder, turn over to the other side and rotate your other arm.

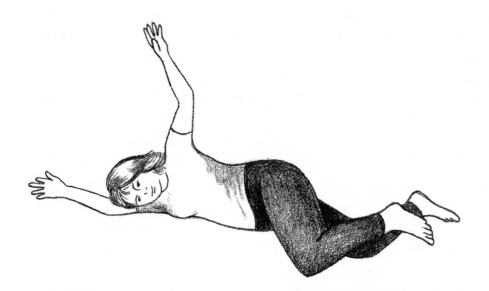

Vacuuming, Sweeping

Vacuuming and sweeping are basically whole-body activities in which the lower body supports the upper body while the upper body maneuvers the vacuum cleaner or broom. It is very important to distribute your weight evenly over your lower body as you move, to stay balanced, to feel the support of your feet and legs, rather than straining your back by lugging your vacuum cleaner from too far a distance across the room. Develop the habit of moving your vacuum cleaner only a short distance, so that your back and shoulders remain comfortable. In fact, it is a good idea to own a lightweight vacuum cleaner that you can pull about easily. Most upright machines are very heavy and require you to push them around from your mid- and lower back, which is very stressful. My vacuum cleaner is a tiny floor model that weighs about five pounds and is easy for me to pull around as I move from room to room.

Because vacuuming and sweeping are such whole-body workouts, it is advisable to do a few exercises before beginning.

SHOULDER CURL. Stand with your feet slightly apart, for a stable base. Let your arms hang loosely at your sides. Your knees are loose, not locked. Feel the crown of your head incline toward the sky. Stretch your arms out straight from your sides, your fingers pointing out straight at the ends of your arms. Relax your shoulders onto your midback muscles. Don't hold your arms up with your shoulder and neck muscles; relax them and feel the support of the muscles in your midback, around your shoulder blades. Next, curl your shoulders up toward your ears. The backs of your shoulders curl up toward your ears and then back down. Twist your wrists as you curl your shoulders. Feel the effects of this motion in your shoulders and back and all along your arms. If you are stiff in your elbows and shoulders, this is an excellent stretch for you. You will feel more comfortable maneuvering a vacuum cleaner or a broom after loosening your shoulders and arms this way.

ARM LIFT OVER HEAD.   Stand with your feet slightly apart, for a stable base. Let your arms hang loosely at your sides. Very slowly, begin to raise your arms so that they will meet, palms together, over your head. Do this extremely slowly so that you can feel each muscle do its part to lift your arms over your head. When your palms meet over your head, hold the position for a breath or two to rest. Lower your arms equally slowly until your hands are back down alongside your hips.

LEG SWING.   Hold on to the back of a chair for support with one hand, while standing perpendicular to the chair (the chair is at your side while you hold on to it with one hand). Begin to swing your inside leg, the one closest to the chair, forward and backward. This should be a loose, easy motion, led by your foot. Your foot swings your leg out from your torso, back and forth. Your straight leg swings out in front of

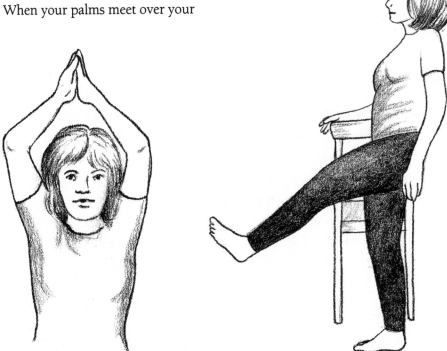

you and out behind you. This swing should not be so vigorous that it affects the straightness of your upper body at all. Let your upper body relax; your legs do all the work.

When your leg is tired of swinging or your supporting leg is tired of supporting, switch sides. Turn around, hold on to the back of the chair with the other hand, and swing the other leg. If your hip joint is very loose and pain-free, your swings will be wide. If your hip joint is tight, your leg won't swing as high. It is important to keep within your own range of motion to loosen the joint.

If this exercise hurts you at all, you might be better off not to swing your leg but to stand on a phone book and let the leg next to the chair just hang from your hip joint. Use your hands to shake the flesh over your hip joint as your leg dangles from it. Breathe and release your leg, so that it feels as if it is falling out of your hip.

LEG SWING TO SIDE.   Hold on to the chair for support, as you did above, and swing your inside leg across your body and then out to the side, then back across your body, instead of swinging your legs forward and back. Let your hips be loose while your foot swings your leg well within your range of motion. When your leg gets tired of swinging or your other leg gets tired of supporting, switch legs and repeat the movement.

WORKING FROM YOUR BODY'S POINT OF VIEW.   When you are ready to begin vacu-uming or sweeping, take the vacuum cleaner or broom loosely in your hands. Let the instrument move in your hands as you work. Because vacuuming is largely a one-sided activity, it is a good idea to change your leading hand occasionally, so that both sides of your body are used. This helps break the common habit of building up one side of the body while the other remains weak and constricted.

As you work, move from your body's point of view. Feel your lower body joints support the movement of your upper body as you manipulate the vacuum cleaner or broom. Focus on distributing your lower body movements over your feet, knees, hips, and lower back. Check the weight distribution on your feet. You should be moving around enough to be shifting your weight so that all your joints—not just a few overworked ones—are moved and share the effort. People with painful ankles and knees tend to plant their bodies in one place and reach everything they can from there. This is a static, inflexible posture that stresses the lower body joints.

If, on the other hand, you are willing to keep moving a little bit at a time, you make a light dancing activity of your work, which gradually loosens and strengthens all the joints of your lower body. It is very important to resist the "freezing" mentality of painful arthritis. The more you introduce movement—gentle, easy movement—to your constricted body, the more possibilities it feels.

Every time you feel your body moving in an easy, pleasurable way, you are increasing the probability that your next movements, too, will be easy. Every time you move in a tense, frozen, reluctant way, you are reducing your options.

Use bending to get under furniture as an exercise, breathing as you curl your spine forward and letting your neck hang loosely forward. If you are sweeping with a broom, let your sweeping motions twist your body gently from side to side and feel the relief in your back and hips as you turn. Let the broom sweep you rather than you sweep the broom. This is a very relaxing attitude and worth the extra time it might take you to clean your house from your body's point of view.

If you tire easily, give yourself permission to stop and rest every few minutes or so. Even if it takes you forever to clean the house, you will feel less pressure if you stop whenever you feel tired. Doing the housework piecemeal may even be a more efficient way to clean it in the long run. Massage your aching parts when you stop to rest. Do any of these exercises that is especially comforting for you. Make yourself a cup of tea to soothe yourself and dramatize the fact that you are making time for yourself.

Making Beds

When we change the coverings on our bed, we enter the realm of the spine. Most of the motions involved in making the bed involve movement of the spine and require a strong, flexible back and associated muscles to perform these motions painlessly. Many people with arthritis or pain of any kind in their backs avoid bending altogether, but this can be a mistake unless there is a particular medical reason not to do so. Curling the back, using every vertebra and its adjacent muscles to support the whole back, is an excellent way to restore strength and flexibility to a stiff back that is weak in some places and overused in others. If you feel your spine stretch, vertebra by vertebra, you activate nonworking areas and relieve overworked areas. So before you start making your bed, do some gentle stretching movements to loosen your spine and get full potential from your back.

SPINE CURL.   This is not a simple "back-bend." In this exercise, you attempt to feel each one of your separate vertebrae as you round your back, lowering your fingers toward your toes. Though such differentiation may seem inconceivable at first, you will find over time and practice that you can distinguish more and more of the separate areas of your back. This accomplishment will indicate that your back is getting much stronger.

From a standing or sitting position, take a deep breath, and on the out-breath let your chin drop toward your chest. With each successive out-breath, push your spine out—vertebra by vertebra—so that your neck is curled, or rounded, and each vertebra is

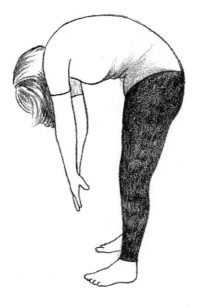

over one of your feet, rather than to the center of your body. Thus you will feel release along your side as well as along your spine. You should place your feet as far apart as is comfortable for you so you will have a broad base of support for this exercise. With each out-breath, you curl another vertebra and drop your arms and head closer toward your foot. After you have curled down as far as you can go, take another deep breath, slowly come up, stand tall for another deep breath, and then begin to curl over the other foot.

REVERSE CURLS. Although it feels great to stretch your spine by curling forward and it is very good for your back, it is also necessary to occasionally curl your spine the other way, in a reverse bow. A very safe and deeply relaxing way to stretch your spine the other way and thereby strengthen the opposing sets of muscles in your back is to slowly and deliberately plant your vertebrae on the floor from a bowed position.

Lie on your back with your knees bent and your feet a comfortable distance apart. Raise your pelvis into the air as high as you can, attempting if possible to get your entire spine off the floor, including your upper body.

Now, breathing regularly, place each vertebra one by one back down on the floor, starting with the vertebra of your neck and upper spine. Even if you cannot do this successfully at first, the effort is important to stretch your spine and strengthen the mus-

stretched as you curl down toward the floor. If you are sitting, your arms dangle toward the floor and your upper body curls until it drapes over your knees. If you are standing, your hands might reach the floor. In this exercise it is important to round the back as much as possible so that each vertebra is stretched away from its neighbors. All the muscles of your spine should support your weight as you bend. So concentrate on "curling up" rather than on merely getting to the floor. The floor is not your goal; stretching your spine is. Feel each vertebra of your spine. After you have done a few curls to the center of your body, try a few to each side.

SIDE SPINE CURLS. These spine curls are performed in exactly the same way as those described above, only on each out-breath you are releasing your head and spine to the side,

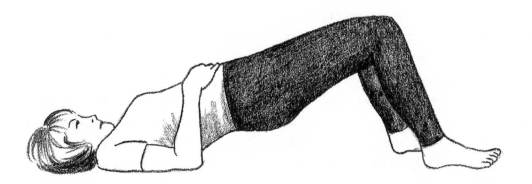

cles that hold it in place. Attempt to lower your spine back onto the floor vertebra by vertebra, as slowly and precisely as you can, until your whole body is back on the floor and you are resting. Repeat again and again until you can feel you have more strength and precision in planting your vertebrae on the floor one by one.

SHOULDER BLADE SWAY IN CHAIR. Sit in a chair facing the back of the chair with legs straddling each side of the chair and hands holding either side of the chair back. Begin to move your upper body from one side to the other, leading with your shoulder blades. As you sway from side to side, feel your shoulder blades shift in your upper back. Allow your sides to stretch slightly with this movement. Do it gently enough that what you feel in your lower back is a slight stretch as you shift your weight, not pain from abrupt movement.

KNEE ROTATIONS WITH FOOT ON CHAIR. Stand in front of a chair facing the seat of the chair. Take a deep breath, and on the out-

breath raise your right foot to the rest of the chair. If a chair seat is too high, use a stool or the rungs of the chair. Put your left hand on your right knee, and begin to rotate your lower leg on the seat of the chair with your hand. Relax your hip muscles, and let your hand lead your knee in rotating motion. Gently beat your right hip with your right

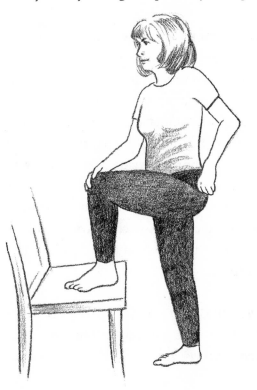

hand or fist to loosen the hip and thigh muscles. Continue until your left leg (the leg supporting you) gets tired. Put your right foot down on the floor.

Take a deep breath, and on the out-breath raise your left leg to the chair, rotate your left knee with your right hand, and gently beat your left hip and thigh with your left hand. Continue alternating legs until the joints in your lower body are relatively pain-free.

You may also massage your ankles, knees, calves, or any part of your lower body with your free hand while the other hand leads the knee in rotating motion. Consider this exercise a combination movement/massage session, and for that reason, it is an excellent antidote for pain.

HIP STRETCH. Stand with your feet apart to give yourself a stable base, and put your hands on your hips. Breathing regularly, begin to slowly move your hips from side to side under your hands, first to the left, then to the right. This is a gentle, stretching motion, not abrupt or vigorous. Use only your hips, not any part of your upper body. Stretch your hips from the left to the right, and feel the gentle stretch in your lower back and inner thighs, depending on which part of you is tight.

WORKING FROM YOUR BODY'S POINT OF VIEW. While you strip the bed and replace the coverings, you can feel the different parts of your spine that need support. Wherever you feel strain and tension, you should become more "active" in your spine, that is, you should curl even more, round your back even more in that area, in order to relieve the strain. The strain comes from putting too much pressure on one particular area of your back. When you curl, or round, your back more and more in that place, you ask more individual vertebrae to share the task of supporting your back, thus relieving the strain too few vertebrae were sharing.

If pulling sheets and blankets off the bed is painful for your wrists and hands, or your fingers, do the pulling with your whole arm as patiently as you can. Feel the effort all the way up your arm starting with your fingers, exerting them the most, then your forearm, upper arm, and shoulder last. If you feel the effort only in your shoulder or upper back, use your lower arm more. This emphasis on an extremity of the body rather than the torso strengthens that extremity and relaxes the torso. Your upper body has the job of maintaining your heart and lungs, regulating your endocrine and nervous systems. You should use your arms to change your bed and leave your upper torso to its other jobs.

It will also be less painful for you if you don't tightly grasp the linens you are pulling off the bed, your hands holding on to them in a clawlike way. Have the patience to weave some ease and flexibility into your chore.

When you strip your bed, place items you

will put back on the bed so that they can be retrieved easily and conveniently. For instance, fold your blanket or quilt so that it can be carried back onto the bed and unfolded in such a way that it spreads over the bed with just a little effort. This is of course much easier on the arms than flapping a heavy blanket or large quilt to get it evenly over the bed. If you treat two or more blankets as one and take them off the bed and replace them on the bed together, you'll also save yourself some trouble.

Large pillowcases are another good idea so that pillows slide in easily.

*   *   *

Although at first it will take a great deal of concentration and patience to break old habits and substitute new ways of moving, you may find when you have been doing your housework this way for a while that not only can you get through it without hurting or straining yourself, but you may even feel energetic enough afterward to do something you truly enjoy. That's what the idea of everyday life as exercise is about: your accomplishing menial physical tasks with energy and spirit. This attitude is crucial for your current vitality and long-term healing.

Chapter 9

Leisure Activities—Good Fun, Good Exercise

People with arthritis often wonder whether specific sports or activities will help or hurt them. Is it okay to bicycle, run, or lift things? They correctly wish to strengthen or restore weak muscles after their joints are loose enough to permit more movement than they are accustomed to, but they wonder how much vigorous motion is safe for them. Indeed, when you have arthritis, too vigorous motion may strain your muscles and hurt your joints. You must focus on your body's sensations to avoid harm.

For example, when you climb on a bike and make that first revolution with your legs, knees, and ankles, you get a feeling about whether you should make one more. If you make one more revolution, you must determine whether to make a third, and so on.

Does this movement make your body feel better or worse? It's not a matter of your head telling your body that you're going to bike ten miles because it's a beautiful day. It's a matter of feeling your joints while you're on that bike. As soon as you feel some tentativeness in your joints or a decrease in your energy level, while you're still on the comfortable side of pain, it's time to turn around and go home.

The length of your exertion is determined by how you feel every moment. If you pay attention most of the time, you can enjoy a ride without hurting yourself. Part of your enjoyment can consist of the very pleasant sensation of your ribs expanding with your breathing, your muscles exerting themselves, and your joints getting looser and looser.

Walking

Walking is well documented as one of the best and least stressful aerobic exercises we can do. And fortunately for many people who would find it a major inconvenience to go to a gym or assemble special equipment whenever they wanted to exercise, walking is so wonderfully available. No special equipment and no investment in clothing or gear are necessary. You can just step outside your door. Of course, it is refreshing to occasionally visit beautiful places that especially relax and inspire you. You can also combine your aerobic exercise period with shopping or errands as long as you keep your priorities straight and do your chores from your body's point of view.

It is especially nice to walk someplace beautiful because you are more inclined to relax and feel your body than when you are also involved in shopping or getting back home in time to finish a task. If you are going to walk for your health and exercise, you must walk in such a way that the expansion and ease of your joints and muscles are encouraged. Walking to get things done in habitual ways that constrict and contract you so that you actually tighten up when you walk is more harmful for you than if you had stayed inside. *How* you walk counts. You want to loosen as you move, to ease tight muscles, to separate joints that are too close together. So you must prepare your body to take a nice long walk, and you must notice what is happening to it while you walk.

When you walk, you need to be aware of the center of your body. If you feel your belly as the center of your body, your stride will be easy and relaxed; your legs will stretch out of your hips, and your shoulders will fall back. Many people unconsciously feel their chest as their center of gravity, and everything operates from there, restricting leg and arm movement, even inhibiting breathing.

Exercises to Make Walking More Beneficial

CENTERING YOUR BODY.   To center yourself, stand with your feet about a foot apart and put your hands on your lower abdomen, your belly. Breathe into your abdomen, slowly and deliberately so that you feel your breath go in and out under your hands. Pat your belly lightly with your open hands to encourage the movement of your breath under your hands. Close your eyes, and feel your moving belly as the center of your universe. Everything falls down around your belly: Your shoulders fall down around it; your vertebrae fall down around it; your legs are mere pillars that connect your belly to the earth. Breathe this way for a few minutes, continuing to pat your belly gently with your hands to emphasize it as the center of your world right this minute.

Then, when you feel quite aware of your

belly, slowly lift your feet in place, one after the other, as you continue to breathe into your belly under your hands. The focus of your consciousness hasn't changed; your belly is still the center of your universe, only now you have added movement in your feet to the sensation you feel in your belly. You can feel your feet moving on the ground, but knowing that your feet are moving does not change your focus on your belly as the center of things. In fact it actually emphasizes that no matter where else movement occurs in your body, your belly does not change; it continues to be the center of your universe as you breathe in and out.

After you have lifted your feet in place for a few minutes without losing your belly as the center of your body, begin to walk very slowly from the same point of view, namely, from your breathing belly as the center of your universe. Your hands continue to feel your belly as it breathes in and out; your belly is still the dominant figure on your internal landscape. Your feet seem to be moving independently, and your body is traveling through space on its own. The fact that your body travels is of no consequence to your belly. Identify with your belly, not with your feet. Stay erect and centered in your belly, no matter how small your steps might be or how altered your usual walk has become in order to accommodate your belly as the center of your body.

WALKING BACKWARD. Now walk backward in the same way, letting your feet and legs feel their way behind you. It may be easier for you to do this exercise than the preceding one, since you have no dominant habit pattern to break as when you are walking forward. It is a good idea to spend some of your walking-as-exercise time walking backward as well as forward. You might try walking backward briefly and walking forward briefly, back and forth, until both ways of walking feel the same. The frustration you feel when first walking backward results

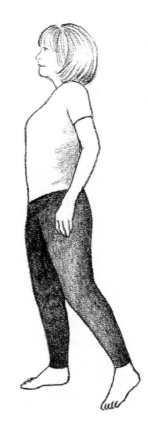

from your not having much previous brain patterning to rely on; your body has to feel its way with each step. This is actually the advantage of walking backward. When you walk backward, your experience of walking—the actual sensations you feel while walking—begins to interfere with your habitual ideas about walking. I have seen people correct long-standing limps by patiently learning to walk backward and allowing that experience to carry over to their forward walk. If you have been limping or walking off-balance for a few months or longer, at least some of your limp is habit.

WALKING SIDEWAYS. Walking sideways is also extremely helpful in breaking bad walking habits, such as limping, leaning forward, favoring one leg, and so on. Begin by standing with feet close together. Put the right leg out to the side and cross over the right foot with the left foot. Continue putting the right leg out and crossing over it with the left leg. After you have walked sideways toward the right for a time, return by using the left leg as the leader and crossing over it with the right leg. Thus both hips have the experience of leading the sideways motion.

KNEES FROM SIDE TO SIDE. Lie on your back with your knees bent and your feet together, your arms comfortably at your sides. Take a deep breath. On the out-breath allow your knees to move your bent legs from side to side. At first you may move just a little bit from side to side. After you feel comfortable with the movement, you can allow your knees to flop all the way to the floor when they move to each side. It is important that your knees lead the motion and that your hips follow rather than the other way around. You are straining your hips in this motion if you can feel the abdominal muscles pull your legs over when you change direction. Feel your knees begin to move before you feel your hips move. That way you can be sure your knees are leading and your hips are relaxing. This is a good preparation for walking because it loosens the hips and alerts the legs to the fact that they will do the work.

KNEES ALTERNATING TO THE MIDDLE. Lie on your back with your knees bent and your feet about a foot apart, your arms comfortably at your sides. Breathe regularly. Allow one of your bent knees to fall between your legs and then return to upright position. Then allow your other knee to fall between your legs and return to its upright position. Continue to alternate your knees to the middle between your legs. This is a good exercise to do along with *knees from side to side,* for the two exercises together stretch the various muscles around your hip joint.

PELVIC CRADLE. Lie on your back with

your knees bent, your feet about a foot apart, and your arms comfortably at your sides. Breathe regularly. Whenever you exhale, flatten your spine against the floor. When you inhale, release and let your spine come back off the floor. Continue to flatten and release your spine as you exhale and inhale, creating a kind of rocking, or cradle feeling.

HAMSTRING STRETCH 1.   Lie on your back with your knees bent. Breathe deeply. On the out-breath, raise one of your legs while keeping it as straight as you can, and with your hands, pull that leg as close to your chest as you can. If you feel a pull in the back of your thigh, rub that area vigorously with one of your hands while the other hand holds your leg toward your chest. Repeat with the other leg.

HAMSTRING STRETCH 2.   Sit on the floor with your legs spread out in front of you. If you have difficulty in this posture—that is, if your knees do not reach the floor and/or you have trouble sitting up straight—put your fist under one of your thighs and push down on your fist with your thigh muscles. Then move your fist to your knee and push down on your fist with the back of your knee. Repeat with the other leg. (If you do not have any difficulty with this posture, go on to *hamstring stretch 3*.)

HAMSTRING STRETCH 3.   If you have no difficulty sitting on the floor with your legs spread out in front of you, you can get even looser with this stretch. What is important is to stretch only on your out-breath so that your breath controls the amount of stretch you do and protects your muscles from injury. Take a deep breath, and on the out-breath place both your hands on one of your

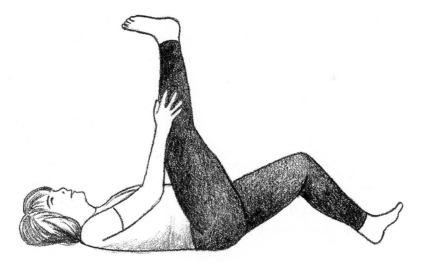

knees. Inhale again, and on the out-breath drop your chin to your chest. Inhale once more, and on the out-breath begin to curl your spine toward your knee. Every time you exhale, allow another of your vertebrae to release your upper body toward your knee. If you reach your knee comfortably, take another deep breath in that position and begin to come up, back to your upright posture. Breathe once in upright posture, and on the next breath begin to curl toward the other knee. Over time you will get loose enough that you can do this exercise with your hands on your feet rather than on your knees. Remember to let this progression happen gradually; there is nothing to be gained by seizing your foot and forcing your body to stretch toward it. You may pull muscle fiber, and you will almost certainly contract your joints. If you are patient and let your body loosen over a period of months, this stretch will benefit your muscles and joints enormously.

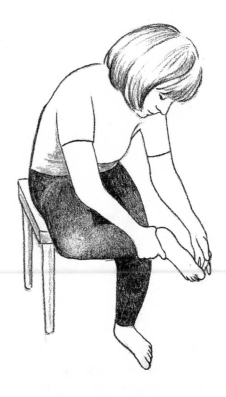

TOE STRENGTHENER. Sit comfortably in a chair, and cross one of your legs over your opposite knee so that you can reach your toes easily. Put one of your fingers under the bottom of your big toe and push your big toe against your finger. Your big toe pushes against the resistance of your finger. Be sure that just your big toe pushes against your finger; don't use your foot, ankle, or any other part of you. You want to use this exercise to strengthen your toes. You will not be strengthening your toes unless you use them exclusively to push against your finger. After your big toe pushes against your finger, move your finger under the bottom of your second toe and push against your finger with your second toe. Continue to move down to the next toe until you have pressed your finger with all your toes, including those on your other foot. Try to press your finger with only one toe at a time, even though there is a tendency for all your toes to press. Do not go on to the next toe until you have succeeded in pressing against your finger with the toe you are touching, even if all your other toes also move.

Now put your finger on top of your big

toe, and push up against your finger. Try to isolate each toe. You may not be able to do this at first, but be patient. In a month or two you will probably be able to move each individual toe, an ability that will bring more movement to your whole foot and have a great effect on your ability to walk in a balanced way.

EXAGGERATED TOE/HEEL WALK. Stand with feet slightly apart. Breathe deeply. Put your right foot as far forward as you can, balancing on your heel. As you bring your left foot forward, roll your right foot forward onto the toes, while your left foot balances on the heel. Roll onto the toes of your left foot while bringing the right foot forward as far as you can. Exaggerate your walk so as to accentuate your putting your weight on your toes and heels.

SPINE CURL WITH ANUS CONTRACTION. Stand with your feet apart and your arms hanging comfortably at your sides. Follow the directions for the spine curl on page 103. When you feel stretched out and curled as far as you can go, begin to contract your anus muscles, the muscles around your sphincter, as if you were trying to prevent a bowel movement. After you have contracted these muscles as hard as you can, contract, or tighten, your buttock muscles as well. You may feel a release in your back as a result of

tightening your anus and buttock muscles and also observe that your hands can go even farther toward the floor.

BALANCE EXERCISE. If you limp, this exercise will help your two sides feel more even. Stand in front of a chair, facing the seat of the chair with your feet apart and your arms hanging comfortably at your sides. Breathe deeply for a few breaths, then on an out-breath lift your foot to the seat of the chair, bending your knee. On the next out-breath, return that foot to the floor and lift your other foot to the seat of the chair. Continue to alternate lifting your feet to the chair every time you exhale. Eventually you will feel as if your two sides are equal in their ability to do this exercise. Then, when you begin to walk again, you will find this equal, balanced feeling continuing into your activity.

Walking from Your Body's Point of View

Now centered, balanced, loosened, and vitalized, you are ready for your walk. Feel your belly as the center of your body. After that feeling is well established in your walking, concentrate on your feet lifting up your legs while your hips and back relax. Feel your arms hang out of your shoulders. Feel your shoulders fall away from your neck. Feel your head stretch up toward the sky.

It is a very good idea to walk on uneven

ground, such as lawn, sand, or gravel. If you walk on pavement, every step you take is the same as the one before. Your feet go on automatic pilot; nothing is stimulated. But if you walk on uneven ground, every step you take is different from the one before, and your feet, ankles, knees, and hips are required to readjust to every new step. Thus your muscles and nerves are activated and adjusting constantly to new stimulation. This is very enlivening and strengthening for your feet and legs. If you live near a beach, that is ideal: You can walk in the wet and the dry sand. If you have no beach or even a park nearby, you can walk on the edge of the lawn. You know you are walking correctly when, at the end of your walk, your calf muscles feel tired but your hips and back feel fine.

If after walking for a while you feel discomfort someplace in your body, stop and fix it with your knowledge of gentle movement and balance exercise. Rotate your hips, rotate your knees; alternately lift your feet to a park bench. Sit down, and curl your spine over your knees. All these movements are antidotes to our tendency to become more rigid as we move. Don't wait until you get home and then collapse. Fix your problem when you have it. Not only will you feel better physically, but you'll realize you're beginning to have some control over the way you feel all the time. You'll have less fear about leaving the house for a day to do errands or for pleasure, because you know that whatever happens, you can do something to make yourself feel better.

When you get home, if you're tired or achy, you can fix yourself a cup of tea, settle onto the couch, and massage your feet and knees for five or so minutes apiece. Or take a hot bath and do some gentle movements in the water, such as bending and straightening your legs against the end of the tub while the warm water supports your legs. Even if you don't feel tired or achy, indulge yourself for your effort. Your body will be grateful.

Swimming Pool Activities

Swimming is the aerobic exercise of choice for people with joint problems because you move through water instead of punishing your joints from the impact of hard ground. I recommend that you make some effort to find a warm pool. Although a cold pool is invigorating and has a very good effect on circulation and swelling, there is a limit to the kind of movements you can do in cold water. For instance, you will want to spend at least some of your pool time doing slow, gentle motions in an unhurried way, and that is very difficult to do in cold water. A warm pool is also the answer to an arthritic's longing for comfort. To find a warm pool in your area, call your local YMCA, ask your rheumatologist or your local chapter of the Arthritis Foundation, or contact the group in your area that tracks resources for handicapped people.

Unfortunately, many people who exercise in the pool do only one or two conventional strokes and don't really make the most of their time in the water to loosen and strengthen all parts of their bodies. Because you are in the water so little of your waking and moving time, it seems a shame not to make the most of your pool session by using parts of your body that you can't use outside of the water. Indeed, you can do many things in the water that you can't do on land. If you have difficulty walking on land with stiff hips, you can stride gracefully through the water with exaggerated huge steps, backward and forward. You can also stretch in the water in ways you can't on land, because you don't have to bear your own weight in the water.

Instead of doing conventional swimming strokes that you have been taught, try experimenting with movements that are tailored to your own particular body. Ask yourself, "Where am I restricted in my movements?" and spend your pool time trying to unlock those areas. Try rotating your arms and legs in all directions, moving your neck from side to side, and bending your spine forward and backward. You'll soon know where you need to loosen up. Concentrate on those particular areas during your time in the water. You'll be working on your body and your particular weaknesses rather than wasting your time on activity that everyone else does.

If you have an hour in the pool, it makes sense to begin your session with small, loosening movements followed by vigorous exercise and then perhaps preparation to leave the pool. (People who have foot and ankle problems will find it painful to carry their own weight again without preparing the lower-body joints to assume it.) Again, as with everything else, you must tune in to your body to make decisions about what kind of exercise you will do in the water that day. When I'm feeling in top form, my pool sessions include ten minutes of gentle warm-up followed by thirty minutes or so of very vigorous swimming or running, followed by twenty minutes of jogging and walking as a cool down. When I'm hurting, I may spend a whole hour floating in a tube and gently moving painful joints from my neck to my ankles.

A few suggestions for exercises follow.

Exercises

FLOATING ON YOUR BACK. Lie on top of the water with limp arms and legs, letting the water around you move your body. Floating is a great way to start your exercise time in the water. First, it is very relaxing. Second, with so little demand on your muscles and joints, you can feel where your particular tensions are and address them specifically when you start to move actively. Third, and perhaps most important, floating without effort introduces a light feeling to your heavy, dense, and painful body. It is very important to your healing that you begin to sense your body as light and flexible again and replace your idea of its being heavy and rigid. Feeling the support of the water with no effort on your part may begin a revolution in your brain. I recommend ten minutes of this experience every time you enter the water.

USING AN INNER TUBE. Put a big tire tube around your neck to float in the water, or place it around your middle to work out your lower body. The latter is a great way to build strength in your legs before your body is strong enough to hold itself up in the water. Even after you are habitually doing more demanding work in the water, putting on a tube after you are tired will help you continue working your legs while the rest of you relaxes. While you are in the tube you can move your legs, feet, and hips any way you like. You can cross your legs over each other in scissor fashion. You can bicycle your way across the pool, leaning back against the tube. You can do a frog kick across the pool, leaning forward in the tube. This kick involves bending your legs out to either side of your body and then moving them out and back to propel yourself forward. If you move your legs out to the side and forward, you propel yourself backward. You should do

both movements in sequence to exercise different muscles in your legs and loosen the connective tissue of your hips.

You can do some serious leg strengthening in the tube by kicking your legs very fast in front of you as you lean back in the tube. If you have a friend to race with in the pool, all the better. There's nothing like a little friendly competition to make you work your hardest. Again, you must confine your efforts to your legs and feet and allow your hips and back to relax. That way, you strengthen your legs and feet while loosening your hips and back.

USING A KICKBOARD. I purchased a little red Styrofoam kickboard so that I could take it with me whenever I visited a pool. I use it to loosen up before doing more vigorous motions in the water and also to work my legs when I am too tired to hold myself up in the water. It allows for more freedom of movement than the tube. The conventional way to use a kickboard is to lie with your stomach on top of the board and kick your way across the pool. However, I find this too hard on the spine for most people, since it compresses the vertebrae in the lower back. It is much more helpful to wrap your arms around the kickboard and hold it in a vertical position as you maneuver your legs in the water. You can bicycle, frog-kick, scissor-kick, and—another advantage over the tube—twist your body in the water while the kickboard holds you up. In other words, you can get quite a bit looser without much effort. On really hard days when I drag my aching body into the pool with no intention of doing anything more than floating and then idly propelling myself up and down the pool on the kickboard, I have often found that after a half hour or so I feel so much looser that I begin to swim the crawl or backstroke.

WALKING IN THE POOL. Walk from one side of the pool to the other, with the water deep enough so that you can walk in ways you would not be able to do on land. That is, you should feel very little impact, and certainly no pain, in your lower body joints.

1. Walk *forward* in the water, raising your legs in an exaggerated fashion, stretching out your legs and hips. Move your arms as well. Come down on your heels when you walk, and push off from your toes in order to loosen your ankles and strengthen the muscles in your lower legs.

2. Walk *backward* in the water, swinging your straight leg behind you, coming down on your toes and falling back on your heels. This should feel like falling backward with each step. Do not lean forward while walking backward. Stay as straight as you can, erring in the direction of falling backward, not forward.

3. Walk *sideways* in the water, swinging the first leg out to your side, then crossing the other leg over the first leg as you move across the pool. Return to the side of the pool where you began so that both legs can experience swinging out, then crossing over.

JOGGING IN THE WATER. Most of us with arthritis can't jog on hard ground, but we can jog in the water. Find a water level (perhaps up to your chin) at which you can jog, that is, propel your body off the floor of the pool by the action of your feet and legs, without feeling any impact in the joints of your lower body. When you find that water level, begin to jog at a comfortable pace, coming down on your heel

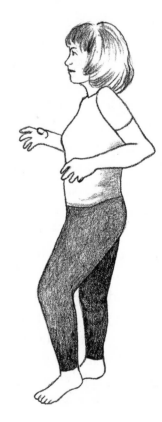

and pushing off on the ball of your foot. This exercises your feet and lower legs in a way they may not be able to enjoy outside of the water when your lower leg and ankle movements may be restricted by pain. By exaggerating the heel/toe movements of your feet in the water while you jog, not only do you get the aerobic benefits of vigorous exertion, but you move your ankle joint in a nonstrenuous way (since there is little weight on it) and thereby build the muscles of your lower leg.

RUNNING IN THE WATER. To run in the water, find a place in the pool where you can freely move your arms and legs without touching the bottom (the water will probably be several inches over your head), and then attempt to keep your head above water by running as fast as you can to keep from sinking. This is a very strenuous exercise and must be built up to gradually. Perhaps you can start out with one minute and then add another minute every few days until you can run in place in the water for five minutes. If you are very out of shape, it is advisable to consult your doctor before you do something this vigorous.

For all of the following water exercises breathe naturally and easily throughout the movements, allowing your diaphragm to expand and shrink with your breath. Check frequently to make sure you are not unconsciously holding your breath during movement.

BENT KNEE FLOATS UP AND FALLS DOWN

1. Stand in the pool with feet about a foot apart so that you feel very stable and balanced in the water. The water should be deep enough that there is little weight on your lower body joints: The water should be at least chest level.

2. Take a deep breath, and on the out-breath let one of your knees float up toward your chest. Your knee is bent, and it slowly floats up toward your chest as you stand on your other leg. Feel the water under your knee support its rise toward your chest.

3. Feel the weight of your raised leg, and let

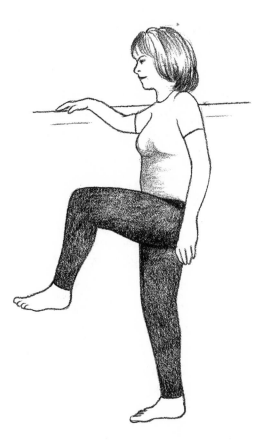

that weight pull your leg back down so that your foot returns to the floor of the pool.

4. Let the other leg float up toward your chest with your knee bent, then let it fall back down.

5. Continue to alternate your knees up and down, breathing regularly and deeply as your knees slowly rise and fall.

ARM SPREAD AND VARIATIONS

1. Stand in the pool with feet about a foot apart so that you feel very stable and balanced in the water. The water should be deep enough that your shoulders are nearly covered.

2. Let your arms float on or near the surface of the water in front of you, your hands near each other.

3. Begin to spread your arms in the water, your open hands leading the motion while your shoulders and arms relax. Feel the water flow through your open fingers while you spread your arms.

4. When your arms reach full spread, release them (let your arm and shoulder muscles totally relax), and let your hands float back to meet each other in front of you again. In fact, if they are very relaxed, your arms will probably cross each other before you exert effort to spread them again.

5. Repeat until your arms and shoulders feel relaxed. Notice the difference in effort between spreading your arms and letting them float back toward each other in the water.

Variations

1. After spreading your arms in the water, instead of letting them float back toward each other, close your hands into fists and bring them up to your chest before spreading them out again.

2. When your arms reach full spread, stretch them just a little farther and hold for a breath before letting them fall back toward each other.

BENT KNEE FLOATS UP, OUT TO THE SIDE, ACROSS THE ABDOMEN, AND BACK DOWN

1. Stand in the pool with feet about a foot apart so that you feel very stable and balanced in the water. The water should be deep enough that there is little weight on your lower body joints: The water should be at least chest level.

2. Let your right leg float up in front of you toward your chest with the knee bent. Feel the support of the water under your knee.

3. When your knee is as close to your chest as it naturally goes when allowed to float in the water, let your bent knee lead your leg out to the side of your body.

4. From the side of your body, let your bent knee lead your leg across your abdomen toward the other side of your body.

5. Feel the weight of your foot and leg, and allow your leg to fall back down through the water until your foot reaches the floor of the pool.

6. Repeat with your left leg.

7. Alternate legs, one after the other, to loosen your hips.

STRAIGHT LEG FLOATS UP, OUT TO THE SIDE, ACROSS THE ABDOMEN, AND BACK DOWN

1. Stand in the pool with feet about a foot apart so that you feel very stable and balanced in the water. The water should be deep enough that there is little weight on your lower body joints: The water should be at least chest level.

2. Let your right leg float up in front of you with your knee extended and your leg straight. Do not make any strenuous effort to keep your leg straight; merely extend your leg in the water, and let it float up toward the surface. Feel the support of the water under your leg.

3. After your leg has floated up in front of you, let your foot lead your leg out to the side of your body.

4. From the side of your body, let your foot lead your leg across your abdomen toward the other side of your body.

5. Feel the weight of your foot and leg, and allow your leg to fall back down through the water until your foot reaches the floor of the pool.

6. Repeat with your left leg.

7. Alternate legs, one after the other, to loosen your hips.

LEG SWINGS

1. Stand in the pool with feet about a foot apart so that you feel very stable and balanced in the water. The water should be deep enough that there is little weight on your lower body joints: The water should be at least chest level.

2. While keeping your upper body straight and stable, and breathing deeply into your abdomen and chest, begin to swing your right leg forward and backward in a slow, rhythmical way. Feel the water against your shin as you swing forward; feel the water against your calf as you swing backward. Feel the stretch in your lower back as you swing forward; feel the compression in your lower back as you swing backward.

3. Repeat with your left leg.

4. Continue until your hips and lower back feel soothed and relaxed.

STRAIGHT LEG TO THE SIDE

1. Stand in the pool with feet about a foot apart so that you feel very stable and balanced in the water. The water should be deep enough that there is little weight on your lower body joints: The water should be at least chest level.

2. While keeping your upper body straight and stable, and breathing deeply into your

abdomen and chest, allow your right foot to guide your right leg straight out to the side at a right angle to your body. This motion should be so effortless that it feels as if your straight leg is floating out to the side.

3. Release your leg, and allow it to float back down to the floor of the pool.

4. Repeat with your left leg.

5. Alternate your legs until your hips feel looser.

BODY TWIST

1. Interlace the fingers of your hands together and drop your arms in the water, allowing your arms to find the place in the water where they are supported without your holding them in place with your muscles. Let your arms float in front of you, held together by your interlaced fingers.

2. Breathe regularly and deeply, and begin to move your arms from side to side, making sure the movement is led by your hands alone. Your hands lead your arms from side to side, changing direction, leading the motion, so that your arms (from the wrists up), shoulders, and neck are perfectly relaxed.

3. Allow your body to follow your hands and arms so that as you move, your body begins to twist from side to side. You might even twist so far that the heel of your foot comes up off the floor of the pool. Feel your body loosen as it gives up to the motion of your arms.

4. Let your head turn from side to side as well, following the motion of your hands and arms.

5. Give yourself up completely to this soothing, very satisfying motion. Listen to your breathing, the sounds in the pool; allow yourself to forget everything except what is present around you and inside you.

6. Continue for several minutes until you are completely relaxed and ready to do something more active.

ON TOES AND HEELS

1. Stand in the pool with feet about a foot apart so that you feel very stable and balanced in the water. The water should be about shoulder level, deep enough that there is little weight on your lower body joints and that your arms will be adequately supported.

2. With your body straight and stable, your arms out at your sides for balance, get up on the very tips of your toes, almost on top of your toenails themselves. If you have difficulty doing this, go into deeper water so you are supported sufficiently.

3. Tighten your knees as tight as you can.

4. Tighten your buttocks as tight as you can.

5. Hold all this tightness for a few breaths, as long as you can.

6. Suddenly release everything all at once: Let your buttocks go; let your knees relax; go from your tiptoes down onto your heels.

Wiggle your toes up in the water with your heels on the floor of the pool. Hang there in the water, enjoying your release.

7. Repeat again and again, alternating between tightness and release.

SCISSORS

1. Hold on to the side of the pool with your legs floating straight out in front of you.

2. Let your feet lead your legs apart horizontally, one to one side and one to the other side, and then bring them together again so that they cross over each other in scissor fashion.

3. Repeat several times to loosen hips.

BICYCLING

1. Hold on to the side of the pool from behind while letting your legs float straight out in front of you.

2. Breathing regularly and deeply, begin to bend and straighten each leg alternately as if you were pedaling a bicycle.

3. Continue for several minutes until your lower body joints feel looser.

FROG KICK

You can do this exercise in two ways: either as you hold on to a kickboard in the middle of the pool or while you are holding on to the side of the pool with your legs floating out behind you.

1. Breathing regularly and deeply, bring both legs up and out to your sides (knees bent), leading with your knees so as not to strain your hips.

2. Straighten both legs simultaneously.

3. Repeat over and over, propelling yourself across the pool if you are on a kickboard, or creating a splash if you are holding on to the side of the pool.

Biking

If you have difficulty walking, riding a bicycle may be a wonderful way for you to feel mobile again, gliding through the countryside, moving in space pleasurably and efficiently, while moving your legs. Biking gives me such a sense of vigor and easy movement, I make it a priority in my week. People are often surprised that although I have trouble walking, I have no trouble biking. The same joints are involved in walking and biking, but you are not carrying your whole body weight on your feet while you are riding a bicycle, nor are your hips and knees sustaining impact with each step. Biking is ideal because you are moving the joints, strengthening your leg muscles, increasing your circulation, and telling your brain how light and mobile you are—all at the same time.

Like any vigorous activity, however, biking can hurt you as well as help you, depending on the way that you do it. Before I became familiar with the vicissitudes of my lower body joints, I went on a bike ride every nice day, taking my cue from the weather rather than from my body. This didn't work very well. Sometimes after I got home I was more swollen in my knees and ankles than when I set out. This obviously was damaging. It became very important to me to learn to know both *when* and *how* to ride my bike.

When to Ride

You need to become familiar with your own body to know what particular energy level and state of being are too low for you to do something so vigorous as taking a bike ride. If I am already a little tired, a little more achy than usual, I'm wise not to get on my bike— and if I must (the day is gorgeous and the flowers are blooming), a couple of blocks will satisfy my yearning to move. You probably shouldn't hop on a bike unless you have a deep, restless, unquenchable *yearning to move*. Vigorous activity is most satisfying when you challenge your body from a sense of feeling restless and confined.

How to Ride

Choose a comfortable bike. Downward racing handlebars are ill-advised, since they require you to bend your upper body over your bike rather than sit up straight. Be sure, for your knees' sake, that you are able to straighten your legs at the bottom of your downward stroke. You should be straight

and tall with no tension in your back or neck as you pedal.

The chief drawback to biking as an exercise for arthritis is that pedaling is so repetitious. If you don't vary the motion, your lower body joints receive the same stimulation and pressure for as long as you ride. Thus, it is up to you to vary the motion as much as you can. The following are the variations I've dreamed up:

At different times during my bike ride, I pedal from three different places in my feet: the ball of my foot, the middle or arch, and the heel. Varying the pressure points in this way enables me to use different muscles in my feet and calves, to stress my ankle and knee joints differently, and to increase my stamina.

I also do various things when I can coast. I pedal backward down hills to relieve the tension in my legs from all that pedaling forward. The most effective thing I do while coasting is hang, or dangle, my legs out of my hip sockets, past my pedals. This stretch has a tremendous and immediate effect on my stamina. I can be quite tired from pedaling up a hill, and this stretch restores me right away. When I ride with people who don't have arthritis, I notice that at first they seem stronger than I—they usually are biking two or three blocks ahead of me as we ride—but they always want to stop and rest before I do, or even to stop for the day when I still have a few good hours left in me. I can only guess that this is because of the way I use my coasting time as a way to relieve tension in my joints and muscles.

I also pay attention to my upper body while riding. People's necks and upper backs tend to get rigid. If you have elbow or wrist difficulties, you will want to shake out your arms occasionally to relieve the tension in those areas. You can relieve neck and shoulder tension by rotating one arm out to the side as you steer with the other. Many times I have returned home with shoulders and neck much looser than when I left.

Perhaps the most important consideration in protecting your joints while you ride your bike is to make sure your legs alone are doing the work and that your hips and back are relaxed. To this end, you must make your body, rather than your biking destination, your priority. When you are climbing a hill, if you can feel your hips and back beginning to join your legs in making the effort to climb, get off your bike and walk it up the hill. Your pedal stroke should always come from your thigh and lower leg muscles. If a hill is too steep for the strength of your legs alone to get you up it without duress to your hip and knee joints, have the sense to get off and walk. Try to ride for pleasure, not endurance.

Warming Up

I suggest that before biking, you give yourself a knee massage (see page 87; massage is good

after biking as well) and then perform the following exercises:

INNER THIGH PULL. Lie on your back with your arms in a comfortable position, the soles of your feet together, and your knees bent out to either side. Now, breathing deeply, begin to slowly, extremely slowly, bring the tips of your knees together at the midline of your body. Move them so slowly that you can feel the extreme pull of your inner thigh muscles as they work to bring your two knees together. When they have come together, drop them again and start over. Continue until you can feel warmth and vitality in the muscles of your inner thigh.

LEG ROTATIONS AROUND HIP. Lie on your back with your knees bent and your feet about a foot apart, your arms comfortably at your sides. Breathe regularly. Now take a deep breath, and on the out-breath lift your right knee toward your chest and take hold of your knee lightly with both hands. Begin to rotate your leg around your right hip joint, allowing your leg to relax as you guide the motion with your hands. Observe how the range of the rotation and the distance of your knee from your chest affect the feeling in your hip. After you have rotated your leg around your right hip for a while, let your right leg go.

Take another deep breath, and lift your

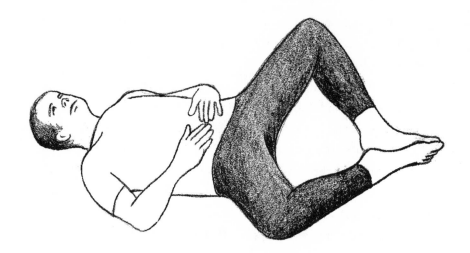

left knee toward your chest, taking hold of your knee lightly with both hands. Begin to rotate your leg around your left hip joint, allowing your leg to relax as you guide the motion with your hands. Be sure to breathe slowly and deeply as you explore the variables of the rotation and the feelings they create in your hips.

LOWER LEG ROTATIONS ON STOMACH. Lie on your stomach with your legs stretched out on the floor. If this position is uncomfortable for you because it compresses your lower back, put a pillow under your hips until your back feels comfortable. If it is uncomfortable because your neck feels strained when turned to one side, put a pillow under your chest so that your neck can hang over

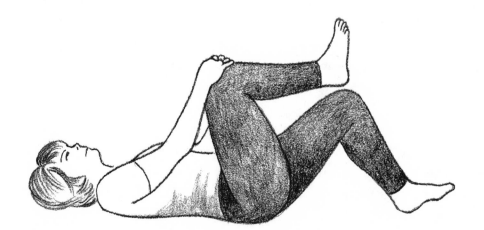

it. Place your arms in a comfortable position, either down at your sides or folded under your head (the latter position may ease your neck strain as well).

Raise your lower legs so that your feet are in the air. Begin to rotate your lower legs around your knees. Relax your hips and lower back so that your feet are leading the motion and your torso can relax. Still, you will feel movement in your hips, especially if your rotations are wide and your lower legs move out to the sides of your body. If this is uncomfortable, make your rotations smaller.

Rotate your lower legs in both directions, feeling as you move the effect the rotations have on your hips and lower back. If you are doing the movement correctly, you should begin to feel some ease in your lower back as you move. If you have been doing it for ten minutes or so and still feel discomfort in your hips or back, stop and visualize your feet leading the motion before you continue again.

If, while you are doing this motion, you notice that one hip feels very different from the other—one draws your attention to it again and again—put one leg down and rotate each leg separately. Finish by rotating the two legs together before you stop the exercise.

Addition. When the rotation of your lower leg is well established, begin to rotate your ankles at the same time so that you are doing two movements at once. This is extremely effective in loosening the whole lower body.

FOOT TO OPPOSITE HAND. Lie on your back with your arms and legs outstretched. Take a deep breath, and on the out-breath your right foot rises off the floor, crosses your body, touches your left hand, then returns to its position on the floor. On the next out-breath, your left foot rises off the floor, crosses your body, touches your right hand, then returns to its position on the floor.

As you get the hang of this movement, begin to do it very rapidly, remembering to lead with each foot, allowing your hips to be pulled by your legs. This is a vigorous hip stretch, done rapidly but rhythmically, and will leave you breathless in a short time. It is fun to do—and extremely effective in loosening the lower body.

This exercise is worth pursuing over time if you cannot do it at first. It is excellent for stiffness in all parts of the lower body and reinforces the message that your upper and lower body can move separately. This message is very important to understand if you are going to ride a bike, because you want to feel the separation between the legs, which are working, and your upper body, which is relaxing. Don't use your upper body when you ride; you will only get tighter and strain your muscles rather than get looser and feel better.

**LEG ROTATIONS IN DIFFERENT DIREC-
TIONS.** Sit back in a chair so as to allow
some distance between your feet and the
floor. If this is difficult because you have long
legs, extend your knees enough to clear the
floor. Rotate your lower legs around your
knees so that your legs are moving together
in the same direction, both of them making
a circle to the right. Change direction, and
rotate both legs to the left.

Separate your knees a little more, and begin to rotate your lower legs in opposite directions so that each leg moves away from
the other as it rotates.

Return to rotating your legs in the same
direction, first to the right and then to the
left, and then repeat the rotation of your legs
in opposite directions. Notice the differences
in ease of movement.

For a final challenge, rotate your ankles at
the same time that you rotate your lower legs
in the same and opposite directions.

LEG STRETCH WITH CHAIR. Stand in front
of a chair facing the seat of the chair. Take a
deep breath, and on the out-breath raise your
right foot to the seat of the chair. When you
have your foot placed on the seat of the chair,
stretch your knee toward the back of the chair
so that the angle between your thigh and lower
leg is decreased. Gently beat your right hip
with your right hand or fist to loosen the hip
and thigh muscles. Be sure to breathe and
stretch within your comfort level. Stretch until

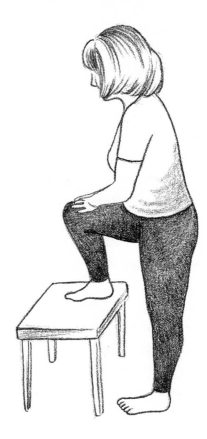

your left leg (the leg supporting you) gets tired.
Put your right foot down on the floor.

Take a deep breath, and on the out-breath
raise your left leg to the chair, and repeat the
stretch and gentle beating motion. Continue
alternating legs until the joints in your lower
body are relatively pain-free.

Watching TV

Watching TV programs or movies on your
VCR is a great time to work on your body,
either with massage or with repetitive movements that would ordinarily bore you.

I like to massage my feet while watching TV. With my mind occupied, my fingers rub gently over the skin of my foot, automatically responding to any swelling or pain they detect. After both feet are done (I continue until I can move the ankles and each toe easily and painlessly), I start on the fingers of each hand. Most people find it hard to massage their hands for a half hour unless they are occupied elsewhere. I find that I can patiently and gently massage each joint of my fingers and hands while I'm being entertained by the antics of some comedian or lover on TV. I'm also willing to massage elbows and knees—anything that ails—when I'm watching TV. I usually devote five minutes to each area, ten minutes to persistently painful areas.

Since most of my TV watching takes place at the end of the day, I go to bed with all my potential trouble spots relaxed and soothed. At first I gave myself a massage only when a part of me hurt me so much I couldn't sleep. But massage before bed turned out to be so incredibly comforting and effective in eliminating the pain for the next morning that I've made it a nightly ritual. (For complete instructions, see the section on self-massage in chapter 6.)

Exercises to Do While Watching TV

MODIFIED BRIDGE.   This exercise is the safest and most comfortable way to stretch your spine in a reverse bow. It can be a tremendous relief for back muscles that have been strained by continually assuming the same posture.

On the floor or a mat on the floor, place a firm round or cylindrical pillow or a bolster under your midback and lie down over it, allowing your head, arms, and shoulders to fall around it. Exactly where to place it is up to you. You should feel a stretch in your chest and shoulders, but it should be quite comfortable. Many people experience a great deal of relief from this posture. If your neck needs support

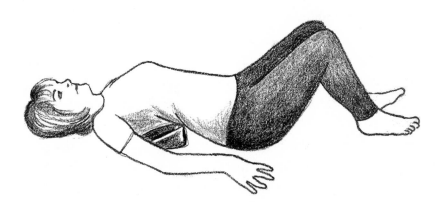

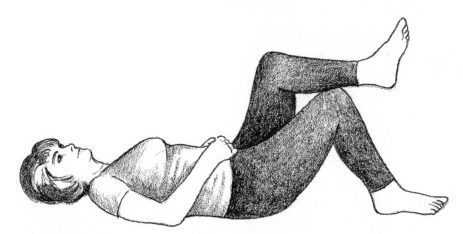

from an additional pillow, use it. Lie in this position breathing deeply for at least five minutes. Move the pillow or bolster a little lower down your back, and try that position as well.

ANKLE ROTATION WITH CALF MASSAGE. If you have stiff or swollen ankles, you should do at least 1,000 ankle turns a day. This exercise combines the ankle turns with a soothing massage of the calves.

Lying comfortably on your back, bend your knees toward the ceiling with your feet together on the floor. Cross your right knee over your left knee so that your left knee supports your right leg right under the right knee. Begin to rotate your right foot around your ankle first in one direction, then the other. Check your breathing and your upper body to make sure your breath is easy and your torso is relaxed.

After your foot rotation is established and easy for you, begin to draw your right calf up and down over your left knee, so as to massage the calf muscles at the same time that

you are using them to rotate your foot. Feel the motion of your calf muscles as you rotate your foot, and massage them particularly where you feel tightness or stiffness.

Lower your right leg, and repeat with the left leg.

Other Spectator Activities

When you're watching a movie, concert, or sporting event in a public place, massage and movement are a little trickier. Nevertheless, they're still worthwhile if you tend to stiffen up while sitting in a restricted position for a few hours. It may be possible for you to rotate your hips slowly and unobtrusively as you sit without being detected. At the very least, you should be able to undulate your spine from top to bottom occasionally. This will keep blood flowing to your legs. You will also be able to massage your fingers while sitting in public. I advise that you rotate your head very slightly on your neck to keep your neck loose whenever you are looking up at a stage or screen.

Exercises to Do While Sitting in a Public Place

The following exercises can be done while sitting in a chair at a lecture or concert, a seat in a theater, a seat or bleacher at a sports arena, and even in a bus or airplane:

KNEES TOGETHER AND APART. Sit on the edge of a chair so that your feet are securely on the ground, your knees together. Begin to pick up your feet, move them out to the sides of the chair, and then back together again. Do this movement rapidly and lightly, loosening up your hips and thighs. Let your feet lead the motion, avoiding the feeling of your hips dragging your legs over to the sides of your chair. Feel that your upper body is relaxed and supported by the chair, and in contrast, your lower body is sprightly and working energetically.

KNEE DIP. Sit on the edge of a chair so that your feet are securely on the ground, your knees together. Move your feet apart as far as is comfortable. With your feet remaining still, allow your knees to fall together in front of you, then move them apart. Continue to alternate dipping your knees toward each other, then moving them apart.

PELVIC ROCK IN CHAIR. Sit in a chair with your feet on the ground. If you like, you can rest your spine on the back of the chair. Put the back of your hand on the last (lower-most) three vertebrae in your lower back. These are the vertebrae you want to move. First relax those vertebrae (slump in the chair), and then contract the muscles around those vertebrae so that your whole upper body is straightened and lifted by the action of these muscles. Don't use *any other* muscles of your upper body. Allow the lower vertebrae of your back to do all the work.

Continue to alternately relax and contract these vertebrae so that you have a fluid, rocking motion in your lower back which lifts and releases your upper body. Do this periodically during the performance or sports event.

HEAD ROTATIONS. Sit in your seat with feet on floor and back supported against the back of the chair. Rest your hands on your knees. Focus your attention on the crown of your head, the area slightly to the rear of the "top" of your head. Feel the crown of your head "reach" toward the sky. Feeling the crown of your head incline toward the sky may cause your chin to shift slightly toward your chest and the back of your neck to stretch almost imperceptibly.

Keeping your attention on the crown of your head, begin to rotate your head in small circles gently around your neck, with the crown of your head leading the motion. It is very important that the crown of your head lead this motion, rather than, say, your chin, because any extreme, abrupt rotation may compress the vertebrae in the back of your neck. By focusing on the crown of your head, you ensure that your backward rotations are subtle and gentle and that your neck is stretched gently forward by your forward rotations.

Change the direction of your rotations from time to time. Take care that you keep the range of your rotations small enough that your head turns loosely and easily on your neck. This way your brain gets the idea that your neck is very loose and your head can turn easily on top of it.

If you do this exercise periodically while watching a movie, you won't get a stiff neck.

LOWER LEG AND ANKLE CIRCLES. Sit in a chair, back far enough so that your feet don't quite reach the floor. (Try the exercise even if your feet still reach the floor.) Begin to rotate your lower legs around your knees, first in one direction, then in another. Let your feet lead this motion, and do it gently enough so that it feels like a pleasant massage for your knees. After your lower leg rotation is well established, begin to rotate your feet around your ankles at the same time, changing direction from time to time. This easy, gentle coordination exercise has the power to loosen the lower body and relax the nervous system simultaneously, making it easier for you to get up after sitting for an extended period.

Chapter 10

Handbook of Exercises

It has been my experience with my own and my clients' joints that usually if one part of the body (the elbow, for example) hurts, you need to loosen another body part (in the case of this example, the shoulder). These exercises have been arranged according to related areas of the body that they primarily loosen, stretch, or strengthen. Conventional physical therapy often focuses on strengthening areas of the body much too soon, before a joint is loose enough to have a full range of motion. This is why I stressed the importance of gentle movements in chapter 4, pp. 42–44. It is important that you read that section before you begin these exercises. Some exercises have appeared in earlier chapters and are cross-referenced here.

Neck, Jaws, Shoulders, and Elbows

In working with your neck, jaw, shoulder, and elbow joints, you are learning to isolate parts of your body that often move as one unit, to your detriment. We tend to use our whole upper body at once, especially when we have lost strength in our fingers and wrists. When you use your shoulder, neck, and upper arm to do something as simple as pick up a cup, rather than just your lower arm and hand, you are contracting your body in an especially vital and vulnerable center. The throat, chest, and neck areas house your respiratory and circulatory centers, as well as various regulatory glands that affect all body functioning.

It is critical to your healing process that you learn to move your head and arms independently of your neck, shoulders, and chest—while driving, working at your desk, cooking, or lifting objects. Optimally, your breathing refreshes your systems while you hoist pots to the stove or move the couch. Your hands and arms apply themselves with great exertion while your shoulders, neck, and chest relax. The emphasis while doing the exercises in this section is best placed on the isolation of the various parts of your upper body, whether you are loosening, stretching, or strengthening your upper body joints.

Loosening

HEAD FROM SIDE TO SIDE

1. Lie on your back with a hard pillow or a phone book under your head. Your arms and legs should be in a comfortable position.

2. Breathe deeply a few times. Then begin to move your head from side to side very slowly and in a way that does not demand anything from the neck muscles. Feel as if someone else has your chin in his hand and is moving your chin from side to side. Stay well within your full range of movement; allow your head to feel very loose at the end of your neck.

3. If there is any part of your neck that feels tense or a little painful, use your hand to tap or rub that area gently at the same time that you continue to move your head from side to side.

4. When your side-to-side movement is well established, add opening and closing your mouth in the same slow, steady rhythm that you move your head. If there is any discomfort below your ears or along your jawline, gently tap the area with your fingertips until the discomfort is eased.

Daily life application: Looking both ways in traffic, turning your head rather than your whole body to look over your shoulder, watching a tennis match or football game, conversing with a person sitting next to you.

ARM ROTATIONS OVER CHEST; see page 70

ELBOW ROTATION; see page 78

STRAIGHT ARM ROTATIONS AROUND SHOULDER; see page 99
Daily life application: Reaching to the side to close the car window, to retrieve a package from the seat beside you, to touch a person or pet beside you.

HEAD ROTATIONS; see page 131
Daily life application: Looking up, looking down, surrendering your neck to the pillow at night.

ELBOW ROTATIONS AROUND SHOULDER; see page 77

UPPER BODY ROTATIONS; see page 72

UPPER BODY DELINEATION; see page 76

Daily life application: Swimming, putting on clothes over head, brushing teeth, shaving face, putting on jewelry or headgear.

ARM ROTATIONS BEHIND BACK; see page 97

ARM SHAKE; see page 92

ARM TWIST; see page 95

ELBOW TWIST; see page 97

HAND SWING; see page 92

Daily life application: Walking with upper body relaxed, draping arm over back of chair, hooking bra, reaching for wallet in back pocket.

Stretching

STRAIGHT ARM LIFT

1. Lie on your back with a hard pillow or phone book under your head. Or you may choose to have no support under your head. Allow your legs to find a comfortable position. Place your arms along the sides of your body, with your hands lying alongside your hips, palms down. Breathe in and out a few times, feeling your abdomen expand and contract with the air.

2. On an out-breath, allow your right hand to lift your straight arm and bring it alongside your head so that your straight arm is lying alongside your head, your hand above your head, palm up.

3. On the next out-breath, your right hand lifts your straight arm into the air and brings it back to lie alongside your hip, palm down.

4. On the next out-breath, repeat with your left hand and arm. It is important to allow your hand to lead the arm motion so that your shoulder may remain perfectly relaxed.

5. Continue to alternate between your two arms. Every time you exhale, your hand lifts your arm into the air and lays it back down.

FINGERS SEEKING OPPOSITE HAND

1. Lie on your back with a hard pillow or phone book under your head. Or you may choose to have no support under your head. Allow your legs to find a comfortable position. Place your arms at a ninety-degree angle to each side of your body, with your palms up. Breathe in and out a few times, feeling your abdomen expand and contract with the air.

2. On an out-breath, allow your right hand to pick up your right arm and lead it across your upper body until your right palm is resting on your left arm.

3. With the fingers of your right hand *(fingers only)*, walk down your left forearm in the direction of your left hand. It doesn't matter if you don't get all the way to your left hand.

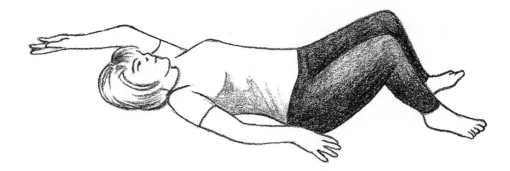

What matters is the stretch in the right shoulder produced by the effort of your fingers to reach your left hand. While your fingers are "walking" down your arm, check to make sure your neck, head, and jaw are relaxed. Only your fingers make the effort in this exercise.

4. When your fingers have gone down your forearm toward your other hand as far as they can, hold the stretch for the length of a complete breath.

5. On the next out-breath, your right hand picks up your right arm and returns it to its former position, at a right angle to your body.

6. On the next out-breath, allow your left hand to pick up your left arm and lead it across your upper body until your left hand is resting on your right arm.

7. Begin to travel down your right forearm toward your right hand with the fingers of your left hand. Make certain only the fingers of your left hand are working and that the rest of your upper body is relaxed and uninvolved in the movement.

8. When your fingers have gone as far as they can go toward your right hand, hold the stretch for the length of a complete breath.

9. Return your left arm to its former position at a right angle to your body.

10. Continue to alternate hands to the opposite forearm.

Daily life application: Reaching objects just out of reach, pulling clothes on upper body, combing hair, drying body with towel, playing golf, swimming.

NECK STRETCH AND KNEE KISS

1. Lie on your back with a hard pillow or phone book under your head. Or you may choose to have no support under your head. Allow your legs to find a comfortable position.

2. Put your hands behind your head and interlace your fingers so that your head is supported by your hands.

3. Take a deep breath, and on the out-breath lift your head *with your hands and arms only* so that your chin inclines toward your chest.

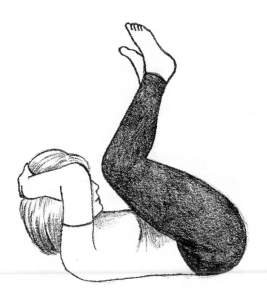

4. Lower your head with your hands and arms, and relax for a breath.

5. Repeat.

6. After you have mastered the neck stretch exercise, try the following variation: At the point where you have lifted your head with your hands so that your chin is touching your chest, lift your knees toward your chest as well.

7. While simultaneously lifting your head with your hands and lifting your knees to your chest with your back muscles, attempt to kiss each one of your knees.

8. Completely release your body, and allow your head and feet to return to the floor.

9. Repeat.

Daily life application: Combing hair, putting on hat or earrings, buttoning or zipping blouse with opening in the back, fastening necklace.

SPINE CURL IN CHAIR; see page 85

TOUCH SHOULDERS WITH FINGERS; see page 92

ARM STRETCH ACROSS TABLE; see page 95
Daily life application: Tying shoes, reaching object on floor, pulling on socks or pants, extending arms in all directions, eating and drinking, applying cosmetics to face, shaving face, reaching shirt buttons, tying tie or scarf.

NECK STRETCH; see page 95

UPPER BODY ROTATIONS WHILE STANDING

1. Stand with your feet slightly apart, for a stable base. Let your arms hang loosely at your sides. Your knees are loose, not locked. Feel the crown of your head incline toward the sky.

2. Put your hands behind your head and interlace the fingers.

3. With your head leading the motion, begin to rotate your upper body at the waist. Your head leads your upper body around your waist. Be careful not to pull your upper body from your lower back; let your head lead this motion. Your head (with your hands and interlaced fingers still behind it) goes

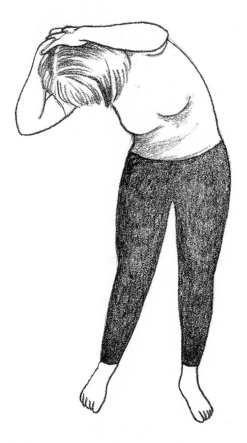

down in front, leading your upper body in a curl toward the floor as it sweeps from left to right or right to left; your head lifts your upper body to an upright position again. Remember to breathe while you do this exercise so that all the parts of your upper body can separate while you move: your head from your neck, your neck from your midback, your midback from your lower back, and all your vertebrae from each other.

4. Change the direction of rotation from time to time.

SHOULDER CURL; see page 100

Daily life application: Tying shoes, pulling on socks and pants, retrieving dropped objects, increasing endurance for desk work, walking straighter.

Strengthening
SHOULDER ROTATIONS ON SIDE

1. Lie on your right side with your right arm either stretched out under your head for support or tucked comfortably under you. You can use a pillow for your head if you like. If it is comfortable for you, bend your upper leg forward so that the knee touches the floor and gives you a great deal of stability. Let your left arm rest alongside your hip.

2. Begin to rotate your left (upper) shoulder. While rotating, encourage your neck to release toward your pillow or supporting arm.

3. Change the direction of rotation from time to time.

4. Turn over and repeat on the other side.

Daily life application: Sleeping better at night, carrying weight on shoulders, carrying shopping bags in hands, pushing or pulling heavy objects.

SHOULDER ROTATIONS; see page 78
Daily life application: Carrying weights on shoulders, carrying bags in hands, pushing or pulling heavy objects.

ARM LIFT OVER HEAD; see page 101

BACKWARD PUSH

1. Stand with your feet slightly apart, for a stable base. Let your arms hang loosely at your sides. Your knees are loose, not locked. Feel the crown of your head incline toward the sky.

2. Straighten your arms alongside your body with your palms facing behind you.

3. Push out behind you with the palms of your hands. After pushing, allow your hands to fall back toward your hips.

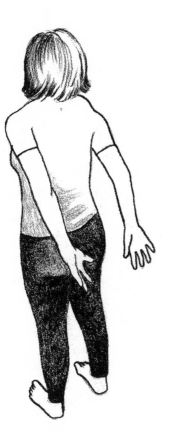

4. Repeat in quick, short motions. Breathe normally during these movements.

CROSS ARMS IN BACK; see page 97

ARM CIRCLES; see page 97

Daily life application: Dressing, washing self, lifting objects, carrying groceries, sweeping, raking, making beds, folding laundry.

Chest, Ribs, and Upper Spine

The chest, ribs, and upper spine are often strained and tight because we get in the habit of using them exclusively instead of other, more appropriate parts of the body that have become too weak. For instance, it is common for people to regulate their walking from the chest and hold themselves up with their upper spine instead of their lower spine if their lower back has become so weak that they no longer feel its support. Not only does this habit strain the upper body and become extremely uncomfortable over time, but the lower spine continues to deteriorate, since it is not used properly. In doing the exercises in this section, you are loosening and stretching your upper body in order to refresh and "rethink" it, that is, to shift the load it carries to your entire spine. Therefore, it is wise to combine your work on this area with various exercises for the pelvis, hips, and lower spine (see following section).

Loosening

ARM ROTATIONS OVER CHEST; see page 70

Daily life application: Pulling clothes over head, washing hair, comfort in sitting, better breathing.

MODIFIED BRIDGE; see page 129

WAVE BREATHING; see page 38

SHOULDER ROTATIONS ON SIDE; see page 138

Daily life application: Better posture, deeper breathing, less strain on neck and shoulders while using arms.

UPPER BODY ROTATIONS; see page 72

UPPER BODY ROTATIONS FACING BACK OF CHAIR

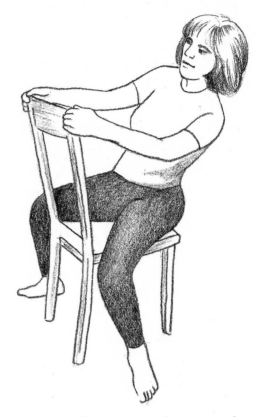

1. Sit facing the back of the chair with your legs straddling each side of the chair. Place your hands on either side of the chair back. Sit close enough to the edge of the chair that your arms are as straight as they can be.

2. Hold on to the chair, and rotate your upper body first in one direction, then in the other. Your chest moves forward toward the back of the chair, then backward away from the back of the chair. Let your arms, shoulders, and neck relax while your chest leads the motion. Make sure your chest moves forward toward the back of the chair before your abdominal muscles take hold. You should try to do this motion without the aid of your abdominal muscles. Let them relax. Your chest and arms are working here. If you feel your abdominal muscles working, relax your hips and legs and make certain your chest moves forward, pulled by your arms, not by your abdomen.

SHOULDER BLADE SWAY IN CHAIR; see page 105

HAND SWING; see page 92

WALL LEAN

1. Stand facing a wall with your feet about three or four steps back from the wall.

2. Put your hands on the wall in front of you, and lean on your hands. Keep your elbows straight. Obviously, this exercise is only for people who don't have difficulty putting weight on their wrists.

3. Begin to shift your weight from one foot to the other, allowing your upper body to move from side to side as you shift your weight.

4. Accentuate the movement in your shoulder blades (your midback area) by pushing your back muscles out against your clothes in the area of your midback.

Daily life application: More comfort while driving and sitting, better circulation in upper body, deeper breathing, support for neck while doing work at desk.

Stretching

LION SHOULDER BLADE STRETCH

1. On your hands and knees, allow your upper spine to sink between your shoulder blades. Let your head fall forward.

2. Shift the weight in your upper body from hand to hand, as lions do. Let all the weight of your upper body hang from your upper spine like a long, self-satisfied cat.

ELBOW FLAP; see page 94

RIB STRETCH; see page 91

Daily life application: Relief from strain of desk work or yard work, better breathing, reaching objects over head.

Strengthening

CHEST STRENGTHENER; see page 39

THROAT MUSCLE STRENGTHENER; see page 39

BREASTBONE FLEX; see page 81

SHOULDER ROTATIONS WITH ARMS IN BACK

1. Sit in a straight chair with your feet planted firmly on the floor in front of you, far enough forward so that it is a slight stretch to put your hands behind you and reach the back of the chair.

2. Put your hands behind you and grasp the two sides of the back of the chair.

3. Holding on to the chair back, begin to rotate your shoulders: first the right one alone; then the left one alone; then both together. Rotate each shoulder in both forward and backward directions.

Daily life application: Lifting objects over head, support of upper spine and neck while sitting and standing, swimming, increasing endurance for house- and yard work, carrying heavy pots, lifting a child, pulling objects across table while sitting.

Pelvis, Hips, and Lower Spine

When the back is healthy, the individual vertebrae are continually moving and stretching in relation to each other in a variety of ways, and all the vertebrae support each other in sharing the burden of your activity, not just a few over and over again. So if you want a healthy back, your spine must become both flexible and strong. The basic movements for the spine in this section involve bending and stretching in various postures and directions to encourage the development of flexibility and strength. The movements in the loosening section can be used to ease a weak, sore back, although there are differences between people. It is very important to do the movements gently and mindfully. A good standard for judging whether you are straining too much is to observe your breathing. If you are breathing easily and even enjoyably, you are pacing yourself correctly. If you find yourself holding your breath or catching it in bursts, you need to do less demanding exercises or to move in a more relaxed and gentle way. If you have any doubts, consult your doctor or therapist.

The key to easing pain and stiffness in the hips lies in (1) developing a loose, strong lower back and (2) loosening and strengthening the muscles and connective tissue of the thigh: inner and outer, front and back. Thus, in doing the exercises in this section, you should give all these areas your attention. You may be surprised at how much easier it is to walk after you have stimulated your inner thigh muscles, an area neglected by most people and often much weaker than the outer thigh muscles. Just as in working on your lower back, it is important to use your breathing as a standard for hip work so that you do not pull any muscles or connective tissue in your hips and thighs.

Loosening

KNEES FROM SIDE TO SIDE; see page 111

KNEES ALTERNATING TO THE MIDDLE; see page 111

LEG ROTATIONS AROUND HIP; see page 125

PELVIC CRADLE; see page 111
Daily life application: Better comfort while sitting or driving, ease in walking, getting in and out of car, changing position in bed.

KNEES OUT AND BACK DOWN

1. Lie on your back with a hard pillow or phone book under your head. Or you may choose to have no support under your head. Allow your arms to find a comfortable position. Stretch your legs out on the floor.

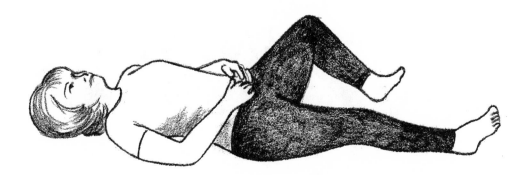

2. Wiggle your toes, and focus on your toes and feet.

3. Take a deep breath, and on the outbreath your right foot moves your right leg up so that it bends your right knee out to the side and then brings it back down to the outstretched position.

4. On the next out-breath, your left foot moves your left leg up so that it bends your left knee out to the side and then brings it back down to the outstretched position.

5. Whenever you exhale, your foot brings your knee out to the side and back down. Continue to alternate legs.

FEET BACK AND FORTH

1. Lie on your back with your knees bent and your feet about a foot apart, your arms comfortably at your sides. Breathe regularly.

2. Begin to bend and straighten your legs alternately as your feet move back and forth on the floor. Put your hands on your abdomen to make certain your feet, not the muscles of your belly, are leading the motion. You can tell if your abdomen is helping in the motion by feeling the movement in your belly. Your belly should feel the same as it does when your legs are not moving.

3. After you are certain that just your feet are doing the motion, speed up the motion until you are doing it very fast, back and forth.

4. Do the motion 100 times, making certain your abdomen is completely relaxed and your breath is regular.

BIG TOE TURN

1. Lie on your back with a hard pillow or phone book under your head. Or you may choose to have no support under your head. Allow your arms to find a comfortable position. Stretch your legs out on the floor.

2. Wiggle your toes, and become aware of your feet.

3. Turn your big toes toward each other, taking care to turn only your feet. Don't use your leg, thigh, or hip muscles. As your big toes turn, they pull your feet along.

4. Release your feet, and let them fall away from each other.

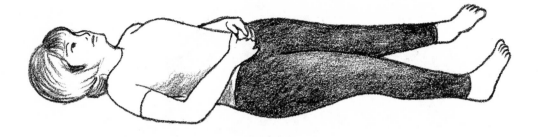

5. Repeat again and again. As you move your big toes toward each other and then release your feet so that they fall away, notice the movement this causes in your hips. Your hips are passively moved (and relaxed) while your feet cause them to turn in the joint.

KNEE IN ALL POSITIONS

1. Lie on your back with a hard pillow or phone book under your head. Or you may choose to have no support under your head. Allow your arms to find a comfortable position. Stretch your legs out on the floor. Breathe regularly.

2. Wiggle your toes, and become aware of your feet.

3. Take a deep breath. On the out-breath, allow your right foot to bring your right leg up so that your right knee is bent and your right foot is on the floor.

4. Move your right knee over to the outside, then move it in toward your other leg (your foot is still on the floor); now your foot brings your knee back down to the outstretched position.

5. Repeat with the other leg.

6. Continue to alternate your legs on your out-breath.

KNEE LIFT TO THE SIDE

1. Lie on your right side, either with your right arm stretched out under your head or with a pillow to support your head and neck. Straighten your bottom (right) leg. Bend your top (left) leg at the knee so that both your left knee and left foot are supported by the floor.

2. Take a deep breath. On the out-breath, lift your left knee toward the sky, keeping your feet on the floor. Only your knee, not your hip or abdomen, lifts your bent leg. Allow your hip and abdomen to relax. Lead the motion with your knee, and let it fall as soon as you feel your hip joint pull your leg, even if you have raised your knee only a few inches.

3. Continue to lift your bent knee on the out-breath.

4. Turn over to the other side and repeat.

KNEE BEND ON THE SIDE

1. Lie on your right side, either with your right arm stretched out under your head or

with a pillow to support your head and neck. Straighten your bottom (right) leg. Bend your top (left) leg at the knee so that both your left knee and foot are supported by the floor.

2. Take a deep breath, and on the out-breath bend your upper (left) knee and straighten it again. Your knee is leading the motion of your leg, bending and straightening, while your hip remains relaxed. If you have difficulty allowing your hip to relax, put your left hand on your knee and focus on the knee's moving your leg. This movement should feel gentle and soothing; it should not be an effort. If you feel effort, focus on your knee as the leader of the movement and move your leg very little, perhaps only a few inches or less.

3. Turn over to the other side and repeat.

LOWER LEG ROTATIONS ON STOMACH; see page 126

LOWER LEG LIFTS

1. This exercise is especially effective as an

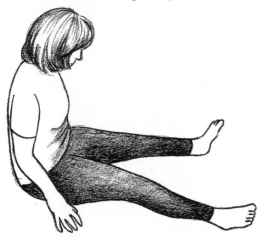

accompaniment to the preceding one, *lower leg rotations on stomach* (see page 126). Do the two exercises together, switching back and forth from one to the other whenever you feel like changing the motion you are doing.

2. Lie on your stomach with your legs stretched out on the floor. If this position is uncomfortable for you because it compresses your lower back, put a pillow under your hips until your back feels comfortable. If it is uncomfortable because your neck feels strained, turned to one side, put a pillow under your chest so that your neck can hang over it. Place your arms in a comfortable position, either down at your sides or folded under your head (the latter position may ease your neck strain as well).

3. Take a deep breath. On the out-breath, lift your right lower leg so that your knee is bent and your foot is in the air. Make certain your foot leads the motion and your hips and lower back are relaxed. If you feel your back working, stop and visualize your foot lifting your lower leg before you resume the movement. In this exercise your lower leg should work hard and your hips and back should be completely relaxed.

4. Lower your right leg, and lift your left one.

5. Continue to alternate lifting and lowering your lower legs.

Daily life application: Relieves pain and discomfort in lower back and hips, enables lower back to support upper body during walking.

LEG SHAKE

1. Sit with legs stretched out in front of you. Do not sit this way unless it is comfortable for you.

2. With your feet beginning the motion, shake your legs from toe to hips as loosely as you can. Your feet turn from left to right and from right to left, and your legs follow, shaking in the hip sockets.

3. If this is a pleasant sensation and doesn't cause discomfort in the hip, continue. If it causes a pressure or pain in the hips, do the *thigh shake*.

THIGH SHAKE; see page 79
Daily life application: Pain relief in hip.

KNEES TOGETHER AND APART; see page 131

KNEE DIP; see page 131

RAISE AND LOWER BENT LEGS; see page 79
Daily life application: Ease in rising from chair, pulling on pants and socks, putting on shoes.

KNEE ROTATIONS WITH FOOT ON CHAIR; see page 105

LEG SWING; see page 101

LEG SWING TO SIDE; see page 102

FOOT TOUCHING STAIR

1. Stand at the bottom of a flight of stairs facing the stairs.

2. Take a breath. On the out-breath, raise your right foot and place it on the bottom stair.

3. Return your right foot to the floor.

4. Take another breath. On the out-breath, raise your right foot and place it on the second stair.

5. Return your right foot to the floor.

6. Take another breath. On the out-breath, raise your right foot and place it on the third stair, and so on until you cannot reach the higher stair.

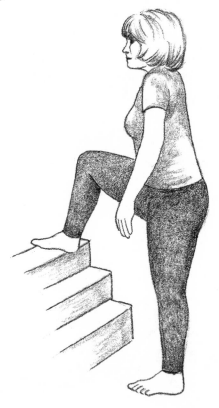

7. Repeat with your left foot.

Daily life application: Correction of limp, ease in walking.

Stretching
STRAIGHT LEGS OVER HEAD (YOGA PLOW)

1. Lie on your back with your knees bent toward the sky and your feet together on the floor.

2. Inhale deeply and exhale. With your hands helping if necessary, lift your lower body, knees leading, off the ground toward your chest.

3. Straighten your legs.

4. Continue to breathe deeply so that areas of your body are released on each out-breath, and allow your feet to drop toward the floor over your head, leading your lower body farther over your upper body so that your spine is stretched.

5. Continue to stretch until your feet touch the floor behind your head. If you cannot stretch that far, stretch only as much as is comfortable. Breathe at least one deep breath in the plow position.

6. Slowly return your lower body to the floor, vertebra by vertebra, breath by breath, so that your spine continues to stretch. Do not just flop back onto the floor abruptly.

7. Repeat.

Modified yoga plow. Follow the preceding instructions, but do not straighten your legs and allow your knees to touch your forehead (rather than stretch out over your head).

FOOT TO OPPOSITE HAND; see page 127

ADDUCTOR STRETCH

1. Lie on your back with the soles of your feet together and your knees bent out to either side.

2. Breathe deeply, and relax your legs as much as you can, allowing your knees to fall toward the floor.

3. Begin to tap your groin area (the area between your inner thigh and your pelvis) with your fingertips to further relax your leg muscles. Continue until your inner thighs have stretched as far as they can comfortably.

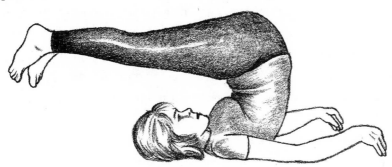

HAMSTRING STRETCH 1; see page 112

LOWER BACK STRETCH

1. Lie on your back with your arms straight out at right angles to your body, your knees bent and your feet together.

2. Take a deep breath, and on the out-breath allow your knees to move your bent legs from side to side. Allow your knees to flop all the way to the floor when they move to each side. In this exercise it is important that your knees lead the motion and that your hips follow, rather than the other way around. You are straining your hips in this motion if you can feel the abdominal muscles pull your legs over when you change direction. Feel your knees begin to move before you feel your hips move. That way, you can be sure your knees are leading and your hips are relaxing.

3. When your knees are flopped all the way to the right, take another deep breath, and on the out-breath allow your left foot (the foot of the upper leg) to bring your left leg (the upper leg) over the right (lower) leg so that your upper leg is stretched across your body. Hold that position for at least a breath.

4. On your next out-breath, your left (upper) foot moves your upper leg back to bent-knee position and you shift your body back to center.

5. On your next out-breath, both knees flop to the left.

6. On your next out-breath, allow your right foot (the foot of the upper leg) to bring your right leg (the upper leg) over the left (lower) leg so that your upper leg is stretched across your body. Hold that position for at least a breath.

7. On your next out-breath, your right (upper) foot moves your upper leg back to bent-knee position, and you shift your body back to center.

8. Repeat the exercise with your other side, this time beating gently with your fist on the stretching muscles of your back, hip, and thigh to loosen them as you stretch.

9. Continue alternating legs and beating the stretching muscles with your fist until your hips and lower back feel looser.

LEG PULL TO CHEST

1. Do the previous exercise, the *lower back stretch*, until you feel very loose and the exercise is easy for you.

2. Now when you cross your upper leg over your lower leg with your out-breath, slip your lower arm under the knee of your upper leg and pull the upper leg to your chest as you exhale again. Hold that position for another breath before you let go and return to center.

3. Repeat with the other side. You can still beat your stretching muscles with your other fist as you pull your upper leg toward your chest. Pull gently; do not force the motion or induce pain.

CAT STRETCH

1. Get on your hands (or elbows) and knees

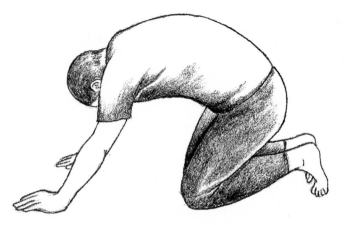

(if this position is comfortable for you; you may want to put a pillow under your knees if they are tender) with your head hanging down in front of you, your arms straight and supporting your upper body, and your buttocks resting on your heels—or as close to them as is comfortable. Breathe regularly.

2. Still continuing to breathe evenly, move your buttocks off your heels and shift your weight onto your hands (or elbows) by moving forward as far as you can. Your lower spine will dip and will be concave or arched. Continue to allow your head and neck to hang as you move.

3. Move back onto your heels. In this position your lower spine is convex, or curved out.

4. Move back toward your heels, and come forward onto your hands. Allow your spine to curve out and curve in alternately, to stretch in both dimensions.

5. Now when you move away from your heels, move your buttocks out toward the right side before you shift your weight onto your hands so that you are moving sideways before you move forward.

6. Now when you move away from your hands back toward your heels, move to the left before you go backward so that you are moving sideways as well as backward.

7. Continue to move to the right from the heels and to the left from the hands so that you are making a wide circular movement instead of just going forward and backward. Change the direction of that circular movement from time to time. Most people find this an extremely pleasant way to stretch the spine in all directions. Make your circular movement as wide as you can without losing your balance. Your buttocks lead the movement, while your upper body relaxes and follows along.

Daily life application: Relief of pain in lower back, ease in standing, wider stride in walking, relief of strain in lower back while walking.

HAMSTRING STRETCH 1; see page 112

HAMSTRING STRETCH 2; see page 112

SPINE CURL IN CHAIR; see page 85

SIDE SPINE CURL OVER KNEES; see page 85

GROIN STRETCH

1. Sit on the edge of a chair so that your left leg is bent normally in sitting posture and your left foot is firmly on the floor. Your right leg, however, hangs over the side of the chair seat (this must be done on a chair without arms). Lower your right knee as far as you can toward the floor, making your right lower leg nearly parallel with the floor. You should feel a stretch in your right groin area.

2. Breathing deeply, exaggerate the stretch in your right groin area by continuing to let your right knee stretch slowly toward the floor. Stretch only on the out-breath.

3. Bring your right leg up, shift position in the chair, and repeat with your left side.

HIP STRETCH; see page 106

SPINE CURL OVER KNEE WITH CHAIR; see page 86

HAMSTRING STRETCH OVER TABLE

1. Stand in front of a table that comes to about hip height. It should be low enough so you can lift one of your legs and easily stretch it across the table.

2. Take a deep breath, and on the out-breath lift your right leg onto the table in front of you.

3. Take another deep breath, and on the out-breath raise your arms over your head and let your chin drop toward your chest. With each successive out-breath, push your spine out, vertebra by vertebra, so that your back is curled, or rounded, and each vertebra is stretched as you curl up toward your right knee. Your head, shoulders, and arms drop toward your knee, and with each out-breath you curl another vertebra and let your upper body fall toward your knee. It is important in this exercise to round the back as much as possible so that each vertebra is stretched away from its neighbors. All the muscles of your spine should in turn support your weight as you bend. Concentrate on "curling up" rather than on merely getting your upper body over your knee.

4. When you have reached your knee, relax in that position for a breath and then come back to standing posture. Put your right foot back on the floor in front of the table.

5. Take a deep breath, and on the out-breath raise your left foot onto the table in front of you and repeat with the left leg.

Daily life application: Bending over to pick something off the floor, weeding, planting, yard work, putting on shoes and socks, washing feet, vacuuming or scrubbing floor, leaning over to a child.

Strengthening

INNER THIGH PULL; see page 125

HIP LIFTS; see page 71

PELVIS ROTATION IN AIR

1. Lie on your back with your knees bent and your feet a comfortable distance apart.

2. Take a deep breath, and on the out-breath raise your pelvis into the air a few inches off the floor, using the quadriceps muscles of the front of your thighs.

3. Begin to rotate your pelvis around your spine, changing direction from time to time. Be careful to use only your thigh muscles to hold your pelvis off the floor. Allow your buttocks and upper body to relax.

REVERSE CURLS; see page 104

INNER THIGH WORKOUT

1. Lie on your back with your arms in a comfortable position and the soles of your feet together with your knees bent out to either side.

2. Take a deep breath, and on the out-breath raise your right leg into the air at a right angle to your body and hold it as straight as you can.

3. Take another deep breath, and on the out-breath slowly lower your right leg out to the right side, parallel to the floor.

4. When your leg is out as far as is comfortable for you, take a deep breath, and on the out-breath your right foot leads your right leg back up into the air at a right angle to your body. It is very important in this exercise that you take care to use *only* your inner thigh (adductor) muscles and not your back or abdominal muscles. Not only will you fail to strengthen your thigh muscles if you use your back or abdomen to lift your out-stretched legs, but you will strain your back or abdominal muscles as well.

5. Lower your right leg, and repeat with the left leg.

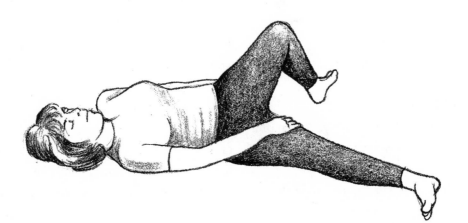

LUMBAR WORKOUT

1. Lie on your right side with your arm or a pillow under your head for support and your bent knees together.

2. Breathe regularly and deeply, and begin to move your lumbar spine slowly in and out, in toward your abdomen, out toward the room. Your lumbar spine should be the only part of your body that moves.

3. Continue alternately stretching and contracting your lumbar spine, allowing the movement to become larger as your body begins to release its tension. You may begin to move the spine laterally as well.

4. Turn on your other side, and repeat the movement.

OUTER THIGH WORKOUT 1

1. Lie on your right side with your arm or a pillow under your head for support and your bent knees together.

2. Straighten your left leg (the upper leg).

3. Take a deep breath, and on the outbreath raise your left straight leg into the air, your foot leading and your hip relaxed.

4. Lower your left leg.

5. Turn over, and repeat with the right leg.

OUTER THIGH WORKOUT 2

1. Lie on your right side with your arm or a pillow under your head for support and your bent knees together.

2. Straighten your left leg (the upper leg).

3. Take a deep breath, and on the outbreath slowly rotate your left straight leg in

the air, your foot leading the motion while your hip stays relaxed. Change the direction of the rotation from time to time. Stop as soon as your leg is tired.

4. Lower your left leg.

5. Turn over, and repeat with the right leg.

TUMMY ROCK

1. Lie on your stomach, and take each foot in each hand behind you so that the only part of you now in contact with the floor is your torso.

2. Begin to rock back and forth from your chest to your pelvis as if you were a cradle.

STRAIGHT LEG ROTATION

1. Sit on the floor with your legs stretched out straight in front of you, your hands on the floor beside you, palms down.

2. With your straight legs together, begin to rotate them in wide circles off the ground. Change direction from time to time. Keep your legs straight and together.

3. Vary the arc of the circles you make with your legs, from large to small. Let your feet lead the motion; allow your abdomen and lower back to relax and feel the strength of your legs.

BACKWARD TILT

1. Sit on the floor with your knees together and bent in front of you, your hands interlaced around the front of your lower legs.

2. Take several deep breaths, and feel the vertebrae in your lower back expand and contract with your breath.

3. Now expand your lower back with your muscles, that is, relax your lower back so that your spine becomes convex—some people call this "slouching."

4. Now, using *only* the muscles of your lower back—not your upper back, not your legs, not your abdomen—pull your lower vertebrae in toward your abdomen. You will feel your spine "rise" as your body becomes straight again. Repeat several times.

5. Let your spine out, and bring your feet off the ground so that you are balancing on your rear end with only your lower back to hold you up. (You may fall over. When you stop falling over, you know that your muscles have become stronger.)

6. Pull your lower back in so that your feet are returned to the ground. Note that just the muscles in your lower back should be doing this work.

7. Repeat several times until you are quite stable in the balancing position and it is only your lower back that is holding you up.

PELVIC ROCK IN CHAIR; see page 131
Daily life application: Stabilize hip joint for greater ease in walking, moving sideways, getting in and out of car, swimming, easing pain in hips or lower back.

Knees, Ankles, and Feet

Arthritic knees benefit not only from knee exercises but also from loosening and strengthening the ankles and feet. That's be-cause the three areas are interrelated. If you can emphasize the toe/heel action when you walk and feel the distribution of your weight over your entire foot, your knees will receive less impact on every step.

Massage is also very helpful for sore knees; you may be able to control any swelling in your knees by gently massaging them every night.

If your feet are the problem, you need support from your lower back, hips, and thighs so that strong muscles help your feet support your weight. If you have ankle or foot problems, it is best to combine the exercises in this section with those in the Pelvis, Hips, and Lower Spine section.

Loosening
KNEE ROTATION IN AIR

1. Lying comfortably on your back, bend your right leg so that you bring your right knee up toward your chest, holding it behind your thigh with your hands.

2. As you hold your leg with your hands, begin to rotate the lower leg around the knee while the upper leg remains in place. Let your foot lead this motion, so that you feel your knee being moved by your lower leg.

3. If your leg can remain in this position for a minute or two without your holding it with your hands, use your hands to massage your knees as your lower leg rotates around it.

4. Lower right leg, and repeat with left leg.

ANKLE ROTATION WITH CALF MASSAGE; see page 130

LOWER LEG AND ANKLE CIRCLES; see page 132

Daily life application: Ease in walking, less pressure on hips, greater distribution of weight on feet, improved circulation while sitting.

FOOT LIFT

1. Stand with feet slightly apart.

2. Begin to lift your feet slightly off the floor, just a few inches, alternating the right and left feet. Bend your knees slightly as you lift your feet. Do this with a loose feeling, so that your knees and ankles have a very slightly bouncy, energetic movement as they lift and fall.

KNEE ROTATIONS WITH FOOT ON CHAIR; see page 105

Stretching

STRAIGHT LEG STRETCH

1. Lie comfortably on your back with your legs stretched out on the floor.

2. Take a deep breath, and on the out-breath lift your right leg toward your chest without bending your knee.

3. As your leg moves toward your chest, help it with your hands. Put them behind your knee and continue the stretch very slowly and gently by pulling your straight leg with your hands.

4. Lower your right leg, relax with a few breaths, and then repeat with your left leg.

HAMSTRING STRETCH 3; see page 112

PARALLEL KNEES

1. Sit on the floor with your legs positioned so that your right knee is bent out to the right and your left knee is also bent toward your right side. Both knees are facing in the same direction about a foot apart. Separate them, but only to a comfortable degree.

2. Put your right hand on your left knee.

3. Put your left hand behind your body and lean on your hand.

4. Take a deep breath, and on the out-breath begin to twist your upper back toward your left arm so that you feel a stretch in your upper back and groin/thigh area. If you do

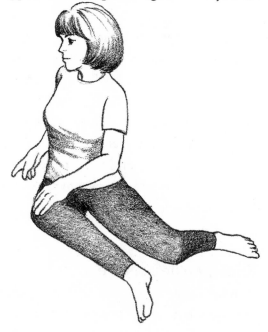

not feel the stretch in your thighs and hips, separate your knees a little farther.

5. Hold this position for a complete breath.

6. On the next out-breath, let your body return to the original position.

7. On the next out-breath, reverse your legs so that both knees face the left side, and repeat with this side. Continue to alternate sides.

ANKLE FLEXION AND EXTENSION; see page 73

ANKLE STRETCH BY HAND

1. While sitting in a chair, cross your leg over the opposite knee, and with your hand stretch your ankle slowly and gently in all positions: toward your shin, away from your shin, toward the outside of your foot, toward the inside of your foot. You can massage your foot and ankle with one hand as you stretch with the other, whenever you feel resistance or pain.

2. Repeat with the other foot.

LEG STRETCH WITH CHAIR; see page 128
Daily life application: Ease of lower back muscles while walking (can reduce pain in lower back if this is present), eases tension in hips, reduces limping, balances gait, distributes weight on feet.

Strengthening
KNEE STRENGTHENER

1. Sit on the edge of a chair so that your back is straight and your knees are bent at the edge of the chair seat.

2. Take a deep breath, and as you breathe out straighten your leg by raising your lower leg to knee level.

3. Release your leg, and let your foot return to the floor, allowing your knee to bend.

4. Repeat with the other leg. Continue to alternate.

ANKLE ROTATIONS; see page 71

TOE STRENGTHENER; see page 113

HIP AND KNEE ROTATIONS; see page 95

TOE/HEEL ROCK; see page 96

EXAGGERATED TOE/HEEL WALK; see page 114
Daily life application: Reduces strain on knees and hips, balances gait, reduces limp, increases ease in walking, sitting, standing.

Hands, Fingers, and Wrists

Perhaps even more than other parts of the body, stiff hands, fingers, and wrists need massage. Both the hand receiving the massage and the hand giving the massage benefit as long as the massage is done gently and without pain. Massage increases strength and flexibility. As with all these exercises, but especially with our hands, we must remember always to keep in mind that the point of the massage is to *feel good*. This means that we will never stretch beyond the point of pain, press hard on inflamed joints, or touch our hands with anything but a soothing, tender stroke. If you follow this massage routine for some weeks, your brain will come to know each of your fingers as distinct from the others, even though you make no conscious attempt to "memorize" the individual characteristics of each one. The combination of the massage and the exercises described below brought my hands and fingers from virtually useless and "deformed" (according to my medical records) to strong, sensitive hands I can use to carry pots, give deep massage, and sew. It is helpful to be very patient and gentle. You may not be able to use a stapler or open a clipboard right away, especially if your fingers have been very stiff for a long time. In that case, it will take some months to regain your function. Be patient and delight in each new discovery of even the tiniest evidence of new flexibility. You may be able to button your shirt before you are able to knit. You will be able to button your shirt and knit before you are able to open tight lids on jars. If you are just beginning to lose the use of your fingers or have lost the use of only one or two, or your ulnar deviation (the tendency of your hand to deviate to the outside because of the deformation of a bone in your wrist) is just beginning to show, you will probably get results fairly quickly. It is very empowering to regain the use of your fingers and hands. You begin to feel as if you are effective in the world again.

Begin by rotating the fingers of your left hand with your right hand. Rotate each finger, including the thumb, in both directions once or twice. These should be easy, gentle rotations, almost, but not as far as, the limit of each finger's ability to rotate. You should stay well within each finger's range because you are loosening your fingers, and it is best in this case to tell your brain how loose and at ease each finger is, not how limited. After you have rotated each finger in both directions, rotate your wrist as well, cradling it gently in your other hand as you move it with your fingers.

Now begin to massage each finger in turn, including the thumb and wrist. This is not a lengthy massage—only a minute or so for each finger—but the massage should be inquiring as well as soothing; that is, the massaging fingers are aware of what they are feeling and where the structures they are feeling disappear or change. The massaging fingers should feel each of the three joints in each finger and all the junctures of possible movement in the wrist. You will notice that some of the joints are relatively flexible, whereas others are swollen, painful, or stiff. Of course, you will favor the most needy joints with your massage.

Next comes gentle stretching of the fingers and then the wrist. Stretch each finger in turn. Gently pull each finger away from the palm of the hand toward the outside of the wrist. You will feel a stretch in the joints of your fingers, more in some joints than in others. If there is a great difference in stretch among the three joints of a particular finger, stretch each joint individually so that some joints are stretched a great deal and others just to the point of pain. Never stretch a painful joint when you feel sharp pain. You may massage a painful joint while you are stretching it and perhaps gain a little distance thereby, but it is not helpful to stress the joints in order to stretch them farther than they willingly go. After you have stretched a finger out away from the palm of the hand, bring the finger back toward the palm and attempt to touch the tip of the finger to the palm. When I did these stretches every day, I usually repeated them until I could touch all my fingers to the palm of my hand. Because my fingers never did this on the first try, I massaged them between stretch attempts until they succeeded in reaching the palm of my hand. This took a great deal of time. I never forced them to get to my palm against pain or stiffness. I always massaged them until they were willing to stretch all the way. To stretch the wrist, take four fingers in your other hand and gently pull them away from the palm of the hand until you can feel the stretch in the front of your wrist. To reverse the stretch, bring the four fingers forward until the tips of the fingers approach the inside of the forearm.

Finish by loosely shaking each finger, thumb, and wrist. Hold each finger by its tip, and shake it gently. Use gentle shaking to impart as much feeling of looseness as you can.

To shake out the wrist, take hold of three or four fingers and shake gently in the same way. You are now ready to do some specific exercises.

EXERCISE SERIES

1. Lie or sit in a comfortable position, and open and close your hands very slowly in an exaggerated way, so that you can feel tiny, subtle bits of motion in the joints and muscles of your fingers. Feel the tips of your fingers as they approach the warmth of your palm, and feel the increasing coolness as they leave your palm. Try this exercise first with both hands. As you become more sensitive, try it with only one hand at a time, then one finger at a time.

2. Lie or sit with your arms at your sides or in your lap, and gently turn your wrists back and forth so that your palms are alternately up, then down. This is a whole-arm movement with the hands leading. Relax your entire arm, and let your hands lead your arms over and back, over and back. Do this motion slowly with exaggerated care so that you can feel exactly how your muscles move your wrists and hands.

3. Lie or sit with your elbows supported on a soft surface, and let your hands lead your forearms in rotation around your elbows. Let your wrists move around your forearms in a limp, relaxed way. If this is painful for your wrists, use your fingers to direct the movement so as to protect your wrists. Focus on

your fingertips, and direct the rotation from there.

4. Sit at a table, and stretch your arms out across it until your arms are straight. Then begin to let your fingertips crawl across the surface of the table, pulling your hands out from the ends of your outstretched arms. Your fingertips should travel as far as they can toward the other end of the table, stretching your hands out from your arms and your arms out from your shoulders.

Daily life application: Manipulating buttons, zippers, shoelaces in dressing; threading needles; writing legibly; playing the piano; eating with regular utensils; brushing teeth and hair with precision; opening stapler removers, clothes hangers with clips; manipulating office equipment like paper clips, clipboards, staplers; changing pen cartridges; turning pages; spreading butter; seasoning dishes in cooking; painting and drawing; signing checks.

Whole-Body Coordination

If you have arthritis or another form of a systemic disease, you might feel that it only makes sense to work on the area that hurts you. The reason I have included a section of exercises that challenge various parts of your body all at once is that moving many parts independently and simultaneously is how your brain learns that your body is loose. It is very important for your body to be loose if you are in the healing process. A loose body moves well and its internal life—the vital organs, glands, and blood—all function optimally to repair and heal the body once they are free of muscular contraction. This is cru-

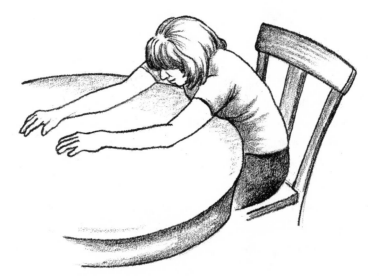

cial to the healing of chronic disease. To do several movements at once while breathing easily and evenly challenges the restrictive patterns of your brain. This kind of healing goes way beyond easing the pain of your shoulder or hip. Over the months it creates new horizons of freedom for your body, turning activities that used to exhaust you into movements you do for pleasure. Many of these movements may be difficult at first, so be patient with yourself. It may take you a while to master them all. Just the attempt itself challenges your brain patterns, so even if you can't do all the movements now, know that just trying is nearly as effective.

UPPER BODY DELINEATION

1. Sit in a comfortable chair with your feet on the floor or on the rungs of the chair. Your back should be supported against the back of the chair. Rest your hands on your knees. Take a few deep breaths and notice the tension in your chest, shoulders, and neck.

2. Put your right hand on your chest, fingers outspread, and begin to gently massage your chest, moving your hand in a small circle over the surface of your skin or shirt. From the point of view of your chest, notice what it feels like to be massaged by your outspread palm and fingers. From the point of view of your hand, notice what it feels like to touch your chest.

3. After the motion of your chest massage is well established, begin to rotate your left shoulder (the shoulder opposite the massaging hand) in small circles, changing direction from time to time, while your left hand continues to rest on your knee or thigh. Feel the distinction between your chest, which is being passively massaged, and your shoulder, which is actively rotating.

4. After your chest massage and shoulder rotation motions are well established, begin to move your head slowly from side to side at the same time, leading the motion with your chin. Move the focus of your attention from chest to shoulder to neck and back again. Enjoy the loose feeling that results from being aware of the distinctions between your upper body parts. Continue to breathe deeply and revel in the independence of your neck, shoulder, chest, and arm.

5. Stop moving and sit quietly for a minute. Notice the difference between the two sides of your upper body.

6. Put your left hand on your chest and repeat with your other side.

Daily life application: Swimming, putting clothes on over head, brushing teeth, shaving face, putting on jewelry or headgear, easing tension in chest, neck, shoulders, watching traffic while driving.

ARMS AND BELLY COORDINATION

1. Sit on the edge of a chair so that your feet are solidly on the floor.

2. Take a deep breath, and on the out-

breath, lift your right arm forward and up alongside your right ear, keeping your arms straight. Be certain that your hand leads this motion so that your shoulder and neck area can relax.

3. Hold your hand up during your inhalation.

4. On the next out-breath, let your right hand lead your right arm back down while you lift your left arm forward and up alongside your left ear.

5. Hold your hand and arm up during your inhalation.

6. On the next out-breath, your left arm comes down while your right arm goes up. Continue to alternate your arms whenever you breathe out.

7. After your arm alternation is well established, continue to breathe normally, and alternately contract and extend your abdominal muscles so that your belly goes in and out while you raise and lower your arms. Feel the independence of your belly and your arms while you move. Continue long enough so that you can easily do the two motions independently at the same time.

Daily life application: Swimming, doing any work involving the hands and arms, like food preparation, desk work, or art work.

SEPARATION OF ARMS AND LEGS

1. Sit on the edge of a chair, your feet solidly on the floor.

2. Take a deep breath. Exhaling, lift your right arm forward and up alongside your right ear, keeping your arm straight. Be certain that your hand leads this motion so that your shoulder and neck area can relax.

3. Hold your hand up as you inhale.

4. On the next out-breath, let your right hand lead your right arm back down while you lift your left arm forward and up alongside your left ear.

5. Hold your hand and arm up as you inhale.

6. On the next out-breath, lower your left arm while you raise your right arm. Continue to alternate your arms whenever you breathe out.

7. When your arm movement is well established, begin to rotate your lower legs around your knees at the same time that you move your arms. Continue to breathe normally. Do the motions so that you feel the independence of your arms and legs—your limbs feel very separated from each other in their movement, and the rest of your body is loose.

8. When your arm and leg motions are well established, rotate your ankles at the same time that you rotate your lower legs. Change direction from time to time.

LEG ROTATION IN DIFFERENT DIRECTIONS

1. Sit back in the chair and lift your feet slightly off the floor.

2. Rotate your lower legs around your knees so that your legs are moving together

in the same direction, both of them making a circle to the right.

3. Change direction and rotate both legs to the left.

4. Separate your knees a little more and begin to rotate your lower legs in opposite directions so that each leg moves away from the other as it rotates.

5. Return to rotating your legs in the same direction, first to the right and then to the left. Repeat the rotation in the opposite direction. Notice the differences in ease of movement.

6. For a final challenge, rotate your ankles while you rotate your lower legs in same and different directions.

ELBOWS, WRISTS, HEAD, PELVIS, KNEES, AND FEET

1. Lie comfortably on your back with your legs spread out on the floor.

2. Bend your elbows so that your hands hang limply at the end of your wrists. Your elbows are supported by the floor.

3. Rotate your lower arms around your elbows very slowly so that you can feel the change in your wrists and lower arm muscles as you do this. Let your fingers lead the motion of your arms around your elbows, which also increases the feeling in the wrists.

4. When the rotation of your elbows is well established, begin to move your head slowly from side to side. Allow your neck to relax completely. Move slowly and gently enough that you don't feel tension in your neck.

Breathe deeply to encourage the separation between the movements of your head and your lower arms.

5. When the movements of your upper body (your head and elbow rotation) are well established, bend your right leg so that the knee goes out to the side, and then move the leg back down so that it is straight.

6. Bend the left leg so that the knee goes out to the side, and then move the leg back down so that it is straight. Be sure you are breathing deeply and evenly. Alternate bending and straightening your legs out to the side while you continue your upper-body movements.

7. Stop alternating your legs. Instead, bend your knees so that they are pointed at the ceiling and your feet are apart.

8. Lift your pelvis into the air and move it to the right, then to the left. Breathe normally and to do your upper-body movements. Try to relax your back so that the main weight of your pelvis is on your thighs.

Daily life application: Ease in using the arms and hands at the same time as walking, such as in operating certain appliances, driving, carrying objects while walking, sculpting, or painting.

CRAWLING

1. Crawl around your room, moving your right arm and right leg forward at the same time and moving your left arm and left leg forward at the same time.

2. Do this movement backward as well.

3. Now crawl around, moving your right arm and left leg forward at the same time, then your left arm and right leg at the same time.

4. Do this movement backward as well.

5. Continue to alternate one-sided crawling with coordinated crawling.

ROLLING

1. Lie on your side with one arm under your head and the other resting on your body. Bend both knees slightly.

2. With the intention of rolling over onto your other shoulder, begin to move your body parts one at a time, rather slowly, beginning with your upper arm. Your upper arm starts the motion, followed by your knees.

3. Turn slowly enough that you expend only the effort necessary to get your body started, and at some point, the weight of your body continues the motion.

4. When you have turned over onto your other side, take a few breaths, relax as long as you need to, and then begin the motion to the other side, again moving your body, part by part, until the weight of your body pulls you over.

5. Continue to roll from side to side, experimenting with leading the motion with different body parts. For example, instead of beginning the motion with your upper arm, try moving only your upper leg until it pulls the rest of you over. Then try starting with your rib cage and so on.

Daily life application: Loosens the entire body, may even enable you to get up from the floor without help if you ordinarily have difficulty doing so.

Index

in treatment of joints, 41
  in water, 64
Muscles, 10, 35, 42, 43, 48, 98

Neck, 7, 17, 44, 86–87, 133–39
Nervous system, 10, 34, 43, 63
Neuropeptides, 13, 27, 50

Osteoarthritis, 62–63
Oxygen, 21, 37

Pain, 3, 4, 5–6, 7, 8, 9, 16–17, 25–26, 55
  attending to, 6, 75
  breathing and, 53
  damage caused by, 54
  with exercise, 42
  exercises for, 62–63
  massage in treatment of, 45, 106
  in movement, 45, 55–57
  sensation and, 52
Pants/slacks, putting on, 79–81
Passive movement, 44, 45, 56–57, 64
Passivity, x, 4, 25
Pelvis, exercises for, 142–53, 161
Personal care, 69–89
Physical work, 59
Physicians, 24, 25, 65, 119
Placebo effect, 27
Plans, planning, 11, 12, 27–28, 52
Pleasure, 21, 25–27, 63–64
Psychoneuroimmunology, 22

Reaching, 90–92
Relationships, nurturing, 21, 27–33
Relaxation, 25, 43–44, 63–64, 88–89, 90
Repetitive movements, 44, 90, 124, 128
Rest periods, 11, 19
Restriction(s), 6, 9, 13, 16–17, 43, 52
  and exercise, 46, 116
  working on, 46, 47–48
Rheumatoid arthritis, ix–x, 3, 8, 21, 26, 90
Ribs, exercises for, 139–42
Rolling, 162
Rotation(s), 44, 56, 70, 71, 76, 77, 156

Schneider, Meir, 5–6, 8
Self-awareness, 46

Self-efficacy, 24–25
Self-healing, 3–9, 25, 26
Self-massage, 86–88
Self-reliance, 69–89
Sensations, awareness of, 51–52, 53, 57–58, 108
Sexual relationships, 32–33
Shaving, 76–77
Shoes and socks/stockings, putting on, 84–86
Shoulders, 17, 44, 133–39
Showering, 74–75
Social relationships, 29–30
Spectator activities, 130–32
Spine, 84–85, 103–5, 106, 139–42
Strengthening exercises, 45, 48, 138–39
  knees, ankles, feet, 155
  pelvis, hips, lower spine, 151–53
  upper body, 141–42
Stretching, 7, 42, 45, 48, 69–70
  fingers, 156–57
  in reaching, 90–91
Stretching exercises
  knees, ankles, feet, 154–55
  pelvis, hips, lower spine, 147–50
  upper body, 135–38, 139–42
Sweaters, putting on, 81–83
Swelling, 10–11, 44, 61, 62, 98, 153
Swimming pool activities, 45, 115–23

Television watching, 128–30
Treatment plan, 61–65

Upper body, 81–83, 106, 125, 133
  exercises for, 134–35, 139–42
Upper body delineation, 76–77, 159

Vacuuming, sweeping, 100–103
Vertebrae, 85, 103–4, 105, 131, 142, 150

Walking, 10, 35, 37, 63, 109–15, 118, 139
Warm pool(s), x, 8, 12, 64, 115–16
Waste products (body), 34, 37, 41, 42, 98
Water exercises, 12, 64
Whole-body coordination, 158–62
Work, 19–20, 57–60
Wrists, 7, 98, 106, 155–58, 161

Zen meditation, 4, 6

Living with Arthritis: Self-Help Morning Workout with Darlene Cohen, the first in a series, is a fifty-five-minute videotape of the gentle movements described in this book for loosening, stretching, and strengthening every joint in lying, sitting, and standing positions.

- Demonstrated by five people with different arthritis difficulties.
- Instruction for individual problems: *what to do when it hurts.*
- Includes *illustrated booklet* explaining each movement.
- It's fun to do your exercises to music with other people on the tape!

Living with Arthritis: Self-help offers you an exercise program that you can safely follow regardless of age or type of arthritis. You begin your session lying in bed, breathing and stretching; then you sit on the edge of the bed to loosen your shoulders, neck, chest, elbows, and wrists; finally, standing with your weight on your lower body, you ease your hips, knees, and ankles. At the end of the workout, you will have moved every joint in your body, increasing circulation to the joints and gently stretching surrounding muscles. You finish by walking with the people on the tape—with a more relaxed, mobile, and energetic body!

To order the videotape, fill out and send in the form below:

Send orders to: HIPBONE PRODUCTIONS
255 Laguna Street
San Francisco, CA 94102

Living with Arthritis: Self-help Morning Workout with Darlene Cohen
    VIDEOTAPE and BOOKLET

_____ copies @ $30.00   _____

California residents: 8½% tax   ---------------

Postage & Handling ($4.00 per tape)   ---------------

                                                Total: _____

BE SURE TO INCLUDE YOUR NAME AND ADDRESS:

Name:_____

Address:_____